AF376701

# Recent Results in Cancer Research 77

Fortschritte der Krebsforschung
Progrès dans les recherches sur le cancer

*Edited by*

*V. G. Allfrey, New York · M. Allgöwer, Basel*
*I. Berenblum, Rehovot · F. Bergel, Jersey*
*J. Bernard, Paris · W. Bernhard, Villejuif*
*N. N. Blokhin, Moskva · H. E. Bock, Tübingen*
*W. Braun, New Brunswick · P. Bucalossi, Milano*
*A. V. Chaklin, Moskva · M. Chorazy, Gliwice*
*G. J. Cunningham, Richmond · G. Della Porta, Milano*
*P. Denoix, Villejuif · R. Dulbecco, La Jolla*
*H. Eagle, New York · R. Eker, Oslo*
*R. A. Good, New York · P. Grabar, Paris*
*R. J. C. Harris, Salisbury · E. Hecker, Heidelberg*
*R. Herbeuval, Vandoeuvre · J. Higginson, Lyon*
*W. C. Hueper, Fort Myers · H. Isliker, Lausanne*
*J. Kieler, Kobenhavn · W. H. Kirsten, Chicago*
*G. Klein, Stockholm · H. Koprowski, Philadelphia*
*L. G. Koss, New York · R. A. Macbeth, Toronto*
*G. Martz, Zürich · G. Mathé, Villejuif*
*O. Mühlbock, Amsterdam · L. J. Old, New York*
*V. R. Potter, Madison · A. B. Sabin, Charleston, S.C.*
*L. Sachs, Rehovot · E. A. Saxén, Helsinki*
*C. G. Schmidt, Essen · S. Spiegelman, New York*
*W. Szybalski, Madison · H. Tagnon, Bruxelles*
*A. Tissières, Genève · E. Uehlinger, Zürich*
*R. W. Wissler, Chicago*

*Editor in Chief: P. Rentchnick, Genève*
*Co-editor: H. J. Senn, St. Gallen*

K.Stanley   J.Stjernswärd   M.Isley

# The Conduct of a Cooperative Clinical Trial

With 9 Figures and 13 Tables

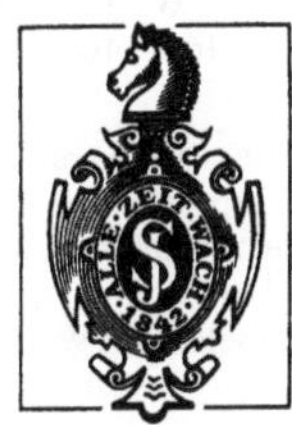

Springer-Verlag
Berlin Heidelberg New York 1981

Kenneth Stanley, Ph.D.
Sidney Farber Cancer Institute, Division of Biostatistics
44 Binney Street, Boston, MA 02115, USA

Jan Stjernswärd, M.D.
Chief, Cancer Unit, World Health Organization (WHO)
Geneva, Switzerland

Mary Isley
Frontier Science and Technology Research
Foundation, Inc., 315 Alberta Drive,
Amherst, NY 14226, USA

*Sponsored by the Swiss League against Cancer*

ISBN-13:978-3-642-81632-1     e-ISBN-13:978-3-642-81630-7
DOI: 10.1007/978-3-642-81630-7

Library of Congress Cataloging in Publication Data. Stanley, K. (Kenneth) The
conduct of a cooperative clinical trial. (Recent results in cancer research : v. 77)
Includes index. 1. Cancer–Therapy–Research. 2. Medical protocols–Standards.
3. Regional medical programs. 4. Medical cooperation. I. Stjernswärd, J. II. Isley,
M. (Mary), 1929–    . III. Title. IV. Series. [DNLM: 1. Clinical trials. W1 RE106P
v.77/W 20.5 S788c] RC261.R35 vol. 77 [RC270.8] 616.99′4s 81-5598 [616.99′406′072]
AACR2



2125/3140–5 4 3 2 1 0

*Preface*

The purpose of this monograph is to address the basic mechanisms for organizing trials. Is is meant to serve as a guide to individuals planning to form a cooperative group as well as to cooperative groups who wish to revise and refine their existing procedures. Current literature deals with many components of conducting clinical trials, such as trial design considerations, randomization, and methods of analysis. But there is a lack of accessible knowledge concerning data flow, data processing, and group organization which causes difficulty for many multi-institutional cooperative trials.

Multi-institutional cooperative studies require greater attention to detail than studies within a single institution. For single institution studies, a single protocol document may be sufficient. In a cooperative group, however, it is necessary to standardize various aspects where little variation may be present in a single institution study. Patients must be entered in a uniform fashion, data collection and evaluation should be standardized, and there must be a mechanism to insure the timely collection of essential data. The Lung Cancer Study Group[1] was chosen as an example to demonstrate the various aspects of clinical trial organization. Standardization in this study is achieved with a protocol, forms, and an operations manual. The operations manual is the heart of the central organization and is given in the following monograph. This manual addresses group organization, an overview of group activities as well as specific mechanics regarding data flow, data management, and quality control. Copies of the protocol and forms are included as appendices. Also included in an appendix is the biostatistical report on the study data available the month that entry onto the study was terminated. This report documents the effectiveness of this trial mechanism.

Although this monograph describes the mechanism under which a well-functioning cancer therapy trial group is operating, the technical procedures detailed should serve as guidelines for cooperative groups in other chronic diseases.

The right ideas, leadership, participants, and long-term economic support are not enough to guarantee the success of a cooperative trial group. An organization must also be devel-

---

1 Footnote see p VI

oped which is able to coordinate the participants and collect and analyze the clinical information.

Biostatisticians and data managers from the Frontier Science and Technology Research Foundation (FSTRF), Boston and Buffalo, were active participants from the very beginning of this study group. Most of the procedures described have been developed by the staff of FSTRF under the direction of Dr. Marvin Zelen. The laboratory, located at the State University of New York at Buffalo from 1971 to 1977, is currently located at the Sidney Farber Cancer Institute, Harvard University, in Boston. The research mechanism detailed in this

---

1 The Ludwig Lung Cancer study group is: J. Stjernswärd, M. Kaufmann (Ludwig Institute for Cancer Research, Inselspital, Bern, Switzerland), M. Zelen, K. Stanley, M. Isley (Frontier Science and Technology Research Foundation, Inc. Boston, MD, USA), C. Mouritzen, P. Paulsen, U. Henriques (Dept. of Thoracic and Cardiovascular Surgery and Institute of Pathology, Aarhus Kommunehospital, Aarhus, Denmark), N. Konietzko, D. Greschuchna, W. Maassen, G. Schubert, W. Wierich, W. Hartung (Ruhrlandklinik and Pathology Institute, Essen-Heidhausen, Germany), D. Oehl (Innere Klinik und Poliklinik, Tumorforschung, Essen, Germany), J. Vogt-Moykopf, D. Zeidler, H. Toomes, W. Doerr, K. Wurster (Thoraxchirurgische Spezial-Klinik und Pathology Institute, Heidelberg-Rohrbach, Germany), F. Krause, R. Rios, R. Spanel (Fachkrankenhaus für Lungen- und Bronchialerkrankungen, Lowenstein, Germany and Pathology Institute, Ulm, Germany), J. Orel, M. Benedik, B. Hrabar, D. Ferluga, T. Rott (Clinical Center, Dept. of Thoracic Surgery and Pathology Institute, Ljubljana, Yugoslavia), P. Lexow (Rikshospitalet, Oslo, Norway), S. Hagen, S. Bugge-Asperhaim, J. T. Stenwig, T. Norman (Ulleval Hospital, Oslo, Norway), T. Harbitz, K. Larsen (Aker Hospital, Oslo, Norway), E. Aspevik, H. Engedal, A. Mykin (Haukeland Sykehus, Bergen, Norway), V. O. Björk, L. Rodriguez, K. Böök, J. Willems (Karolinska Sjukhuset, Thoracic Clinic and Pathology Dept., Stockholm, Sweden), E. Grädel, J. Hasse, P. Holbro, P. Dalquen (Kantonsspital, Chir. Dept Thoraxchir. Klinik and Pathology Institute, Basel, Switzerland), L. Eckmann, K. Hänni (Tiefenauspital, Chir. Univ. Klinik, Bern, Switzerland), B. Nachbur, H. U. Würsten, H. Cottier, A. Zimmermann (Inselspital, Dept. of Thoracic and Cardiovascular Surgery and Pathology Institute, Bern, Switzerland), W. Maurer, M. Kaufmann, P. Froelicher (Bürgerspital, Surgical Dept., Solothurn, Switzerland), H. Denck, St. Wuketich, E. Zwintz (Krankenhaus der Stadt Wien-Lainz, I. Chirurgische Abteilung and Pathol.-Anatom. und Bakteriol. Inst., Vienna, Austria), N. Pridun (Pulmonisches Zentrum der Stadt Wien, Vienna, Austria), K. Karrer (Institute for Cancer Research, Vienna, Austria), H. Hackl (Patholog.-Bakteriol. Institut am Psychiatrischen KH der Stadt Wien, Vienna, Austria), H. Holzner (Pathology Inst., Vienna, Austria), D. S. Freestone, R. Bomford, M. T. Scott, T. Priestman (The Wellcome Research Laboratories, Beckenham, England)

monograph is based on procedures developed over many years by this laboratory in its collaboration with numerous cooperative groups, including the Eastern Cooperative Oncology Group, the Radiation Therapy Oncology Group, the Working Party for Therapy of Lung Cancer, and the Veterans Administration Lung Group.

One of the most reliable verifications that a particular intervention is effective is by a randomized controlled clinical trial. This is true especially in the area of cancer therapy. Institutions have realized that a collective research effort is needed in order to carry out definitive therapeutic trials. It is our hope that the material in this monograph will be helpful in this respect.

Kenneth Stanley
May 1981

# Contents

Contents                                                          XI

# 1 General Organization

## 1.1 Introduction and Objectives

We have an ethical obligation to search for better therapies for most types of cancer. A cooperative study group offers the opportunity for oncologists to answer scientific questions that lie beyond the capability of a single institution. The objectives are to define sound medical hypotheses, develop and execute the investigations that will provide answers to the hypotheses, and thereby improve cancer treatment and patient care.

Work in a cooperative group should be done according to the principle of "one for all and all for one". No one individual should be identified more than the others and publications should be authored under the group name. This principle has been found important for gaining full collaboration of all the participants. If a chairman publishes the joint effort of the group under his name and some selected collaborators, the enthusiasm and input of patients may be less than if the above principle is followed carefully.

A meeting between the participants before starting the trial is important. Not only the clinicians but also individuals from other key disciplines should participate in this meeting and be included as full members of the study group from the start. For example, the inclusion of the pathologists is essential. When creating a clinical study group for trials in a disease, biologic research should be planned from the beginning. The costs for this are relatively small in comparison with the overall costs. New biologic information is likely to result even if the treatment modalities investigated show no therapeutic benefit.

Some general principles to be fulfilled in a clinical trial are:

1) Sufficient patient accrual. Participation from enough centers should be guaranteed before starting so that we can both stratify *and* treat according to prognostic subgroups. This is to avoid overtreatment and undertreatment, permitting therapy to be designed according to identifiable biologic subgroups.
2) Accrual should take only 2 years. If not, other therapies may appear, proven or not, that may make it ethically difficult to continue. Further, accrual itself often drops due to diminishing enthusiasm.
3) The trial should be designed so that conclusive results, whether positive or negative, will be achieved.
4) New information on the biology of the disease should be sought – not only a comparison of therapies.
5) To realize the above principles efforts have to be pooled. Single small trials are often a waste of resources.

The purpose of this monograph is to describe the mechanism of a cooperative clinical trial. The first study of the Lung Cancer Study Group has been chosen to illustrate these principles and procedures. The objectives of this randomized study are to explore whether intrapleural immunotherapy by *Corynebacterium parvum*

(*C. parvum*) can increase recurrence-free interval and survival in operable patients with bronchial carcinoma and to identify high risk patients after identifying biologic prognostic factors (see the study protocol, Appendix 1). A Phase I study exploring the feasibility of giving (*C. parvum*) intrapleurally was undertaken before the radomized study began [11].


## 1.2 General Organization

Twelve institutions participated in this study, situated in four central European countries and three Scandinavian countries. The Coordinating Center is in Bern, Switzerland, and the Statistical Center is in Boston, Massachusetts. With good organization and sufficient economic support, an intercountry or intercontinental clinical trial group is not much more difficult to run than an intrainstitutional study. A number of the common terms used are defined in Appendix 11.


## 1.3 The Coordinating Center

The coordinating center is the administrative headquarters for the Study. It comprises two components, the administrative office and the operations office. The responsibilities of the administrative office are to:
 1) Suggest and design studies,
 2) Arrange meetings and find participants,
 3) Raise economic support,
 4) Disperse funds,
 5) Synchronize the clinical institutions, statistical center, and operations office,
 6) Plan future studies,
 7) Review institution participation in conjunction with the statistical center,
 8) Prepare and disperse periodic accrual reports and circular letters,
 9) Coordinate review procedures for material proposed for publication,
10) Coordinate any future protocol for review by participants and statistical center.

The responsibilities of the operations office include:
 1) Operation and control of the central randomization desk,
 2) Collection of patient forms,
 3) Distribution of forms to the study coordinator and the statistical center,
 4) Maintaining patient files for the study coordinator,
 5) Distribution of computerized requests and study status lists from the statistical center to participating institutions,
 6) Monitoring of the institutions' response to computerized requests,
 7) Distribution of final record reviews,
 8) Reproduction and dissemination of biostatistical reports,
 9) Inventory of forms, replenishing institution's supply when requested and notifying the statistical office of additional printing requirements,
10) Distribution of protocols.

## 1.4 The Statistical Center

The two key individuals at the statistical center are the statistician and the data manager. It is the responsibility of the statistician to use his professional skills at all stages of the study. These include:
1) Study design,
2) Protocol and forms development,
3) Patient randomization,
4) Implementation and supervision of data management,
5) Statistical analyses, both interim and final,
6) Collaboration in preparation of presentations and publications.

It is the role of the statistical center data manager to:
1) Assist the statistician in the design of the study, protocol, forms, and data processing plan.
2) Maintain the integrity of the study by:
   a) Reviewing forms and clarifying questionable data with investigators through the use of clarification requests;
   b) Identifying problem areas of interpretation in the protocol or forms;
   c) Discussing with the statistician any problem areas such as serious reactions to treatment;
   d) Soliciting decisions from the study coordinator on questions of eligibility and protocol interpretation and adherence.
3) Initiate the computer files by coordinating the efforts required of the data entry operator, programmer, and data base administrator.
4) Maintain and update the existing computer files.
5) Monitor the accuracy of data entry.
6) Prepare the operations office logs, and the participants and statistical center portion of the group Operations Manual.
7) Plan and present data management workshops for the participant data managers.
8) Schedule and prepare the patient listings (every 2 months) and the forms requests (3 months before a meeting).
9) Inform the study coordinator of problem areas such as:
   a) Which institutions are negligent in sending data;
   b) Recurring errors in data submission which should be brought to the attention of all the investigators.
10) Periodically send computer listings and reports to the study coordinator to assist him in monitoring the studies.

# 2 Overview of Group Activities

## 2.1 Introduction

The conduct of a clinical trial occurs in three phases. In the first phase the study is conceived, the protocol and forms are designed, and the data flow and processing plans are prepared. In the second phase the study is actively accruing patients. Patients are entered, forms are completed and reviewed, and interim reports are prepared. The data flow is assisted with data requests and status lists. The third phase begins after patient entry is terminated. All patients are followed-up until death and the data flow and review continues. During this phase definitive analyses will be prepared upon which group publications will be based.

## 2.2 Protocol Generation

The initiation of a new study is accomplished as follows:
1) The initial conception of the study takes place at a meeting of participants.
2) A preliminary draft is prepared by the coordinating center and statistician.
3) This preliminary draft is circulated for review among the participants.
4) Comments are collected and discussed and an initial version is prepared. (The actual protocol is printed in yellow so that it is not confused with the drafts printed on white paper.)
5) As the situation warrants, a review of the protocol is undertaken, suggested revisions discussed, and a revised version prepared.

## 2.3 Forms Generation

The forms required to collect and record data for a study evolve in the following manner:
1) The end points and data important to the study are discussed by the study coordinator and statistician.
2) A preliminary draft is drawn up by the statistician and the form is computer generated.
3) The data base administrator and study data manager review the forms and make suggestions; revisions are made by computer.
4) The revised form is sent to the study coordinator for his comments and for circulation among the investigators.
5) Suggestions are reviewed by the study coordinator and statistician.
6) Revisions are made on the computer and reviewed by the data base administrator and study data manager.
7) A final copy is sent to the printer.
8) As the situation warrants, a review of the forms is undertaken, suggested revisions discussed, and a revised version proposed (as in steps 5−7 above).

## 2.4 Patient Entry

Patient entry is centralized and coordinated through the operations office. To enter patients, the investigator telephones the operations office. During the telephone conversation, eligibility will be verified and the stratification factor (type of surgery) will be recorded. The treatment assigned to that patient and a number for study identification purposes are given to the investigator.

Once a case is entered on study a Confirmation of Registration Form is completed by the operations office and sent to the investigator and the statistical center. This form serves three purposes:

1) It is a verification of the phone registration, giving protocol criteria and assigned treatment.
2) It becomes the first record for the computer file for that case, and is the basis of all future reference to the case.
3) It confirms the patient's randomization number which should be used on all future correspondence.

## 2.5 Data Flow

The flow of information is given schematically in Fig. 1.

## 2.6 Form Submission

All data are submitted on standardized three-part NCR (no copy required) forms. Participants should complete the form, remove the last copy, and send the remaining two copies to the operations office. The operations office logs the form, removes the second copy for filing, and sends the top copy to the statistical center.

Standardization of criteria is assisted by the forms; standardized criteria for clinical staging, surgical staging, and toxicity are found on the reverse side of the appropriate form. Other standardizations such as eligibility, end point definition, treatment administration, patient monitoring, and patient management are given in the protocol.

## 2.7 Completed Forms Review

All submitted forms are reviewed by the statistical center data manager for completeness, consistency, and protocol adherence.

Data queries or clarification of inconsistent reporting are mailed routinely from the statistical center to the institutions as the data is reviewed. Replies should be sent to the operations office.

## 2.8 Computerized Requests and Status Lists

The purpose of the forms request is to obtain the most current data possible while the status list is generated for information purposes. Examples are given in Appendices 3 and 4.

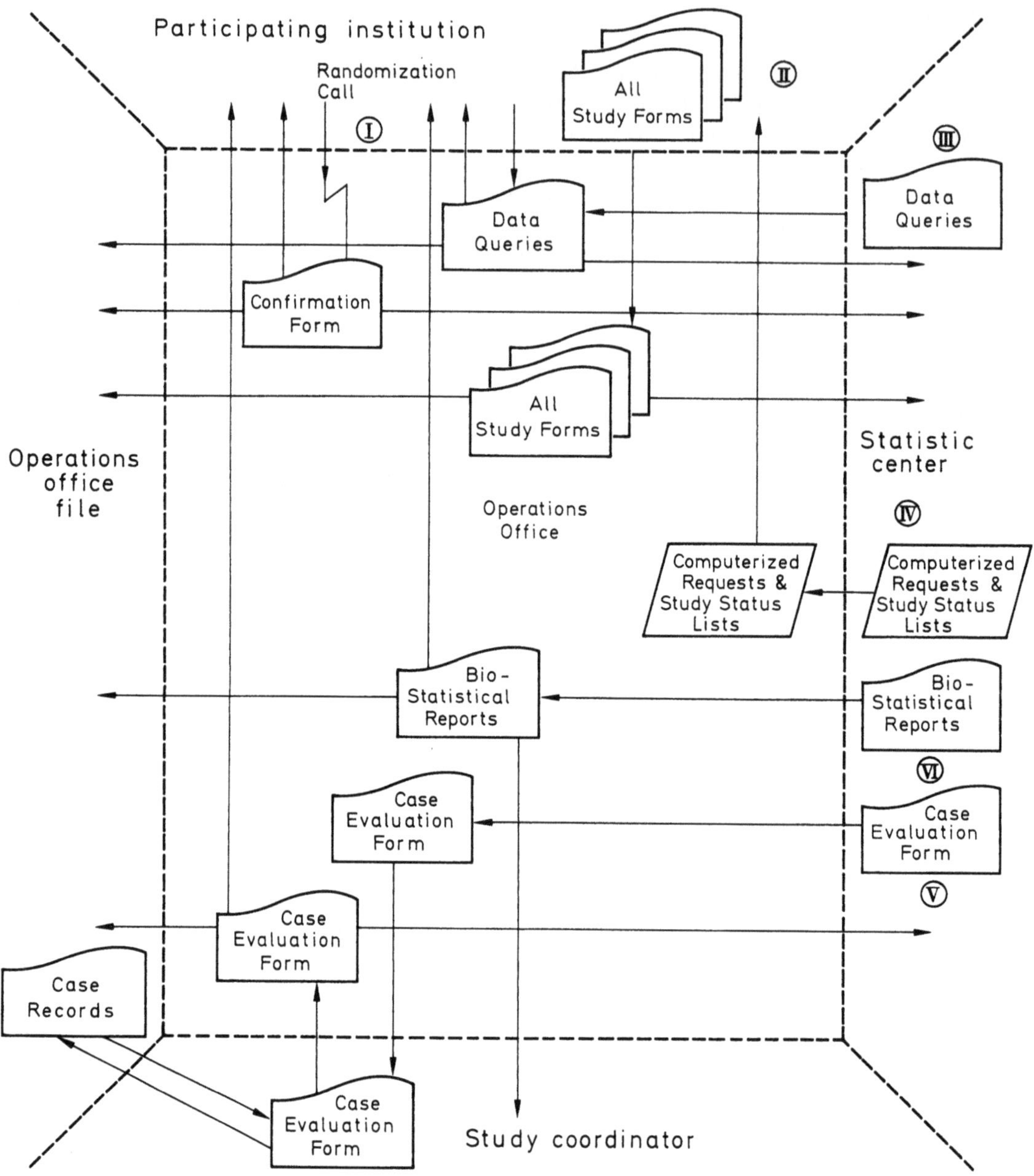
Participating institution
Randomization Call
I
All Study Forms
II
III
Data Queries
Data Queries
Confirmation Form
All Study Forms
Operations office file
Operations Office
Statistic center
IV
Computerized Requests & Study Status Lists
Computerized Requests & Study Status Lists
Bio-Statistical Reports
Bio-Statistical Reports
VI
Case Evaluation Form
Case Evaluation Form
V
Case Evaluation Form
Case Records
Case Evaluation Form
Study coordinator

Computerized lists reporting the current clinical status of the patients, the current status of the patient's records, and requests for missing information from each institution are sent to the operations office by the statistical center. The operations office forwards them to the participating institution.

The operations office maintains a copy for the computerized request lists and monitors the response from the institutions, contacting them if necessary. Responses to a computerized listing should consist of forms which are to be processed in the usual fashion.

## 2.9 Records Review

Patient records are reviewed by the study coordinator at three points in time:
1) Eligibility is reviewed as soon as sufficient forms are available.
2) First recurrence is reviewed as soon as it is reported.
3) The major end points are reviewed when patient death is reported.

Review of eligibility is conducted by the V1 form. The V2 form (not finalized yet) is used for the remaining record review. In all cases the statistical center data manager will initiate the record reviews. The appropriate review form is completed and sent to the operations office. At the operations office the study coordinator reviews the case and denotes the result of the review on the form. When the review has been completed the top copy of the form is returned to the statistical center for file change, if necessary, a copy is sent to the institution that entered the patient, and a copy filed at the operations office. When the final evaluation is entered on the computer, the record processing is considered completed.

## 2.10 Biostatistical Reports

Biostatistical reports are prepared by the statistical center for group members at approximately 6-month intervals. Preliminary reports stress patient entry, data flow, treatment administration, and complications. Subsequent reports address the primary end points (an example is given in Appendix 10). The biostatistical reports form the basis of group publications of the trial results.

**Fig. 1.** Stages in the flow of information in the clinical trial. *I* Participating institutions call the operations office to randomize a patient. The operations office prepares the Confirmation Form, retains a copy for their file, sends one copy to the institution, and sends the original to the statistical center. *II* All study forms are completed by the institution and sent to the operations office where one copy is retained for their file and the original is sent to the statistical center. *III* The statistical center sends queries about forms to the institutions via the operations office. Replies are routed the same way. Copies of responses to queries are filed at the operations office. *IV* Computerized requests and study status lists are sent by the statistical center to the operations office where they are separated and forwarded to the appropriate institution and a copy filed. *V* The Case Evaluation Form is prepared at the statistical center and reviewed by the study coordinator along with all forms. He enters his comments and judgements on the Case Evaluation Form. It is then distributed by the operations office to the statistical center and the contributing institution. One copy is filed at the operations office. *VI* Biostatistical reports are sent by the statistical center to the operations office for reproduction and dissemination

# 3 Institution Specific Activities

## 3.1 Institutional Data Management

Each participating center designates a data manager. This individual is responsible for submitting all study forms, responding to all data and clarification requests, and telephoning for patient entry. Specialization of this responsibility promotes efficient data collection leading to high quality therapy evaluation. A keen appreciation for organization of medical information is most essential. Participation in a training session conducted by the statistical center, known as a data management workshop, is highly recommended.

## 3.2 Patient Entry

When it is decided to place a patient on study, the eligibility requirements in the protocol should be reviewed. This will indicate the information that is needed to randomize the patient. A careful review of available patient information should prevent the entry of an ineligible patient.

The participant should call the operations office and answer the eligibility questions. The name of the member hospital from which the patient is being entered will be given as will the other necessary information (randomization criteria and stratification factor, i.e., type of primary resection). It is helpful to spell out the patient's name, as subsequent forms have frequently shown the name to be incorrect. The clinical sequence number should also be recorded during the phone conversation. The clinical sequence number is the identification number assigned to the patient in each hospital. The treatment and randomization number will be assigned by the operations office and a confirmation form will be sent.

## 3.3 Forms Submission

All patients should be followed-up until death. Patients found to be ineligible after entry in the study must still be followed.

Forms are to be submitted as listed in the protocol. All forms are sent to the operations office for distribution. The bottom (pink) copy of each form should be torn off prior to submission and filed. This copy is for the participant's records. It is suggested that the participants maintain the patient records in the same fashion as the operations office and statistical center. There should be a folder for each patient's record. These folders should be ordered by randomization number and identified with the patient's randomization number, patient name, and clinic sequence number.

It is recommended that the data manager have a forms submission log listing all study patients from the institution. This would be correlated with whatever means is used for scheduling appointments for follow-up visits. An example is given in Appendix 5.

Each form contains instructions for its completion and the required time for submission. There should be no blanks on the forms. If data is unobtainable, this should be noted. Examples of the forms are given in Appendix 2.

### 3.3.1 Clinical and Preoperative Form B

Form B contains information concerning the patient's disease prior to resection. It should be accompanied by Form F (first column only). Form B confirms certain eligibility requirements of the protocol. Note the use of "−1" for unknown items. The following points should be noted about questions (Q.1−Q.34) in Form B.

*Q.1.* The patient should not be more than 70 years of age.

*Q.4.* Surface area should be given to establish dose relationship. Refer to Appendix 1.3 for the surface area chart.

*Q.6.* Note that a bone marrow biopsy should be performed if a weight loss of 10 kg has occurred within 6 months (see "Parameters" section of the protocol).

*Q.7−Q.13.* A "2" (yes) answer indicates the patient is ineligible.

*Q.14−Q.16.* If the flow sheet (Form F) for the period prior to surgery shows liver enzymes to be suspect for liver metastasis, one of these tests should have been performed and proven negative.

*Q.19.* If mediastinoscopy is positive, the patient is ineligible.

*Q.20.* See Q.6.

*Q.21−Q.30.* Distant metastases make the patient ineligible.

*Q.31−Q.34.* The staging definition appears on the reverse side of the form. Any stage greater than 2 would make the patient ineligible.

### 3.3.2 Surgery Form C

This form is to be completed after surgery.

*Q.2. Type of Resection.* The answer should be consistent with Confirmation Form A. If not, this should be explained in the comments section. Surgery other than standard resections will make the patient ineligible.

*Q.4−Q.13. Involvement by Site.* If answered "2" (yes) these items should be compared to Form D for histologic proof.

*Q.15. Location of Primary Tumor.* The codes should be consistent with Q.2.

*Q.16. Size of Primary Tumor.* Measurements are to be rounded off to the nearest centimeter.

### 3.3.3 Histology and Study Treatment Form D

This form is to be completed after pathologic examination of surgical specimens and administration of *C. parvum* or placebo. It should be accompanied by Form F (column 3 only).

*Q.2, Q.3, Q.4, Q.8, Q.9, Q.10, Q.14.* If answered "2", the patient is ineligible. A response of "3" (not investigated) is the proper answer if there has been no histologic examination. Any site noted as involved on Form C should not be answered "3" or "9" on Form D.

*Q.14.* If Form C indicates no pleural effusion, the answer to this question should be "9" (unknown).

*Q.15–Q.18.* Staging definitions appear on the reverse side of the form. Any stage greater than 2 makes the patient ineligible.

*Q.19. Histologic Classification.* This should not be small cell carcinoma.

*Q.21.* The date of administration must be after the date of randomization and should be before the tenth day postoperatively. Any delay must be explained. If there is a delay between removal of draining tubes and administration, the reason should be noted.

*Q.22.* Administered dose should be 7.0 mg, if no modification occurred. Some have been incorrectly reported as 0.7 mg; this would indicate 7/10 not 7.

*Q.24.* This refers to the insertion of the catheter at time of surgery as stated in the "Treatment Administration" section of the protocol.

*Q.25.* Any modification should be explained in detail; additional sheets should be used if necessary. If placebo was not administered, this question should be answered "4" (treatment not administered).

### 3.3.4 Follow-up Form E

This form is to be submitted every 3 months for the first 3 years, commencing 3 months after surgery and must be accompanied by flow sheets (Form F). After the first 3 years, the submission schedule is every 6 months. At the time of death, Form Z must also be submitted.

*Q.1–Q.2 Follow-up Time Period.* Each form should follow the previous Form E with no time period unaccounted for. If any change in the status of disease is noted, Form E should be submitted immediately although it may not be scheduled until later.

*Q.3.* Any answer other than "1" (no evidence of disease) requires an explanation in Q.4–Q.7. The explanation may be one or more events.

*Q.4.* Question 4 is the most important section on any form, as the time to recurrence is the primary end point of the study. It is necessary to specify the *site* of recurrence and the method of detection. Form E is the only report of disease progression by site at the time of relapse.

*Q.8–Q.11. Additional Therapy During This Report Period.* If answered "2", the details should include: (a) the reason for therapy if not related to events in Q.4–Q.7; (b) for surgery the date, type, and site of surgery; (c) for radiation therapy the inclusive dates, dose, field, and reason for administration (e.g., respiratory complications); (d) for chemotherapy the dates administered (from, to), agent, dose, frequency of administration (e.g., daily X 2 weeks, monthly from 1/12/77 to present) and reason for administration; and (e) any other pertinent data, including dates.

*Q.12–Q.19.* In the event of death, Q.12–Q.19 should be completed. Contributing factors, Q.14–Q.18, should be answered individually, not left blank. There may be more than one contributing factor. If cause of death is other than protocol disease, Q.3 should indicate the status of protocol disease. Q.3 should not be left blank.

Occasionally, a patient may be lost to follow-up. This may be due to a move to another country or location. Every effort should be made to follow-up the patient, but if that fails, "lost to follow-up" may be reported. The incidence of lost to follow-up on this study should be slight, as geographic suitability is an eligibility requirement.

### 3.3.5 Flow Sheet Form F

This form is to be completed whenever the patient is examined at the institution. It is the form which will be used most frequently. If tests have not been performed at given timepoints, this form should be submitted with the notation indicated.
Once study treatment is completed, the flow sheets may be sent in with the follow-up form, but there should be a flow sheet for each visit.

### Prior to Surgery

It is especially important that column 1 of this form be completed prior to surgery. This is necessary to provide the data prior to treatment in order to assess the effects of treatment. Ignorance of a preexisting condition could prejudice the evaluation of treatment.

### Subsequent Forms

It is necessary to record the results of the required tests at the timepoints specified and each time the patient is seen: column 2 within 24 h prior to administration of *C. parvum* or placebo; column 3 between 24 and 48 h after administration of *C. parvum* or placebo; and column 4 at all other times.
*Q.1.* The date should be completed on all submissions.
*Q.2–Q.10.* In several cases, study requirements have not been met. If tests are not performed, "−1" should be entered in the last two boxes on the right for each test, e.g., $\boxed{\phantom{nn}\phantom{nn}\phantom{n}|-|1}$ WBC. For hematology entries, actual values should be used (these should not be reported as "normal"), e.g., WBC 7,800, platelets 179,000.
*Q.11–Q. 15.* In several cases, study requirements have not been met. If the prerandomization flow sheet reports abnormal liver enzymes, Form B will be checked for additional tests. If abnormal liver enzymes are attributable to other causes, this should be noted on the form.
*Q.16–Q.22.* Any abnormality which is present initially should be noted.
The prerandomization flow sheet in comparison with subsequent flow sheets is the basis for evaluation of treatment-related complications. To achieve a standard reporting of data, the chart given on the reverse side of Form F should be used.
*Q.23.* Performance status should be reported when indicated, using the Karnofsky Scale, which is printed on the reverse side of the flow sheet.
*Q.24.* The clinical investigation should be reported when indicated on the flow sheet.
*Q.25.* The lung X-ray should be reported when indicated. If not performed, a code of "9" should be entered.

### 3.3.6 Death Report

Forms E and Z should be submitted at time of death.

### Forms in Developmental Stage

*Pathology Forms.* These forms are under discussion by the pathologists. A preliminary version of Form P, the pathology form, is given in Appendix 2. It is anticipated that these forms will be completed by the pathologist.

*Central Pathology Review Form.* This form, Form R, is currently being developed. It will record the result of central pathology review on material submitted to the operations office. The most recent version of this form is included in Appendix 2.
*Death Report.* Once finalized, this form will be completed retrospectively. A preliminary version of the autopsy form, Form Z, is given in Appendix 2.


## 3.4 Clarification Requests

When the statistical center data manager detects an error, questionable entry, missing information, or inconsistency on a form, a request for clarification is sent to the investigator, via the operations office. Responses to these requests should be sent to the operations office in the usual fashion.


## 3.5 Computerized Requests and Status Lists

Periodically, computerized requests for forms are sent to the investigators, via the operations office. An example is given in Appendix 3. These requests indicate a date of required submission. Information received at the operations office by this date is guaranteed processing and analysis in the next biostatistician's report.
If a form is requested which was submitted within the previous 4 weeks, this request should be disregarded as that allows mail and processing time; if it was submitted earlier, a photo copy should be mailed.
A major change in a patient's status should be reported immediately. This information should not be delayed until the next scheduled report.
If a particular assessment or follow-up is not performed, this fact should be reported. If only a portion of the information is available, this data may still be valuable. If the forms request lists a follow-up on a particular date, and the patient was not seen or heard from close to that time, this fact should be reported and the closest available information submitted.
Patient status lists giving basic patient data are circulated periodically. These lists are broken down by institution and are ordered by randomization number and alphabetically. An example is given in Appendix 4. These lists are to provide the status of a participant's patients at a glance. If any information is incorrect, the statistical center should be notified, via the operations office.

# 4 Coordinating Center Specific Activities

## 4.1 The Administrative Office

The administrative office maintains the group's administrative files. These files include group correspondence involving protocol, forms and manuscript development, and group participation as well as economic matters. This office maintains an up-to-date mailing list of the group membership for group communication purposes. Monthly circular letters are sent to all participants giving accrual by month and participant, plus any necessary group communication. An example might read as follows:

Enclosed please find the interim report on the progress of our trial No. 1. Warmest thanks are owed to you all for so efficiently submitting the data and to the Statistical Headquarters for a detailed Biostatician's Report.

Prognostic factors are emerging and high-risk patients may be identifiable for future trials. This is just as or even more important than the outcome of the therapies compared. To make a definitive interim report in the summer of 1979, we need as soon as possible:

a) all outstanding forms (see enclosed data request, Appendix 3);

b) all remaining pathology slides/blocks (these should be sent to the coordinating center);

c) complete pathology forms.

Encl.: Biostatician's Report, February 1979 (see Appendix 10).

Monthly accrual chart (see Fig. 2).

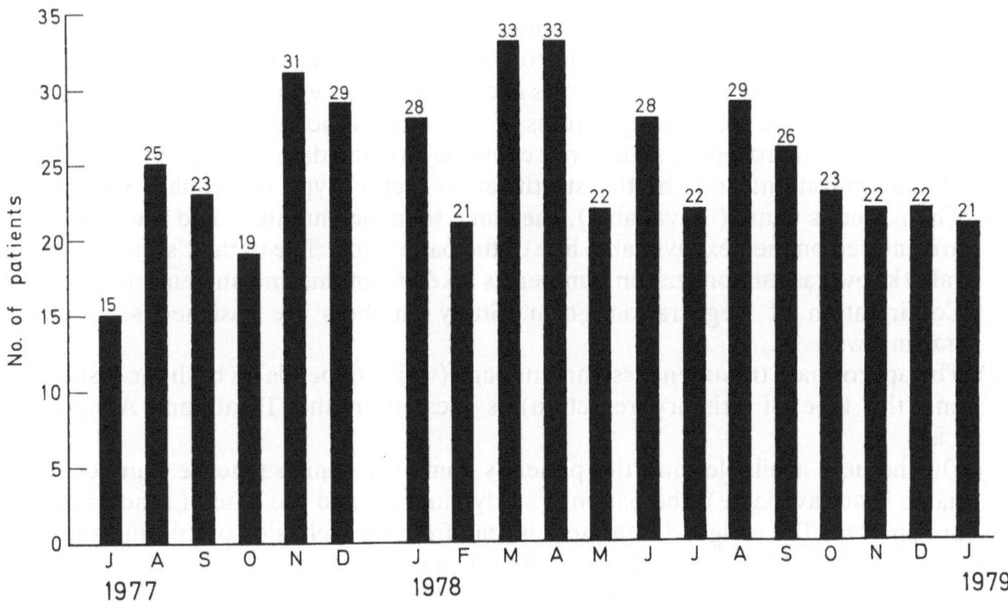


**Fig. 2.** Entry of patients per month into Trial I

## 4.2 Patient Entry

The operations office performs the randomization of patients into the trial. Randomization materials are provided by the statistical center.

### 4.2.1 Material

The necessary material for registration and randomization consists of:
1) *Confirmation of Registration Forms* (Form A), which are used to record telephoned randomization information and also serve as a confirmation to the institution of the treatment assigned over the telephone.
2) *Treatment Assignment Lists*, which are computer generated and contain the randomly sequenced treatments to be assigned. These lists are ordered by hospital and by stratification factor (type of primary resection) within each hospital. A sample page is given in Appendix 7.
3) The *Patient Log*, from which patient numbers are assigned sequentially as patients are entered onto the study and on which the receipt of subsequent forms is entered. An example is given in Appendix 6.

### 4.2.2 The Randomization Procedure

When a telephone call is received for the purpose of randomization, the individual at the operations office responsible for the randomizations (called the registrar) will utilize the following procedure:
1) A blank Confirmation Form is selected (Form A).
2) Onto this form are entered: (a) the name of the institution; (b) the person calling; (c) the patient's name (if the institution is willing to provide it); (d) the clinic sequence number (an institution identification number assigned to that patient; if the number is too long for the boxes provided, the entire number is written on the sheet next to the boxes and the last digits entered into the boxes); (e) the answers to the eligibility questions (if the patient is not eligible for the study, the randomization procedure should not continue); (f) the date of surgery; (g) the date of randomization; and (h) the stratification factor (type of primary resection).
3) The patient's name (if available), the clinic sequence number, and the institution are entered on the next available line of the patient log. The patient's study number (also known as randomization number) is taken from this line and entered onto the Confirmation of Registration Form. Study numbers are assigned sequentially starting with 1.
4) The appropriate treatment assignment page (which depends on both the institution and the type of primary resection) is located in the Treatment Assignment List.
5) On the next available line, the patient's name (or clinic sequence number if the name is not available), the patient's study number, and the date of randomization are entered. The assigned treatment is read from the right side of this line and then entered onto the Confirmation of Registration Form.
6) At this time, the caller is notified of both the treatment that has been assigned, and the study number for that patient which will be used on all future correspondence.

The treatment, not the code for it, is relayed verbally. The phone connection can be terminated at this time.

7) Next, the "follow-up forms are due" section is completed. To fill in this section, the registrar only needs to write down the dates of 3-month increments, the first of which is 3 months after the date of surgery. For example, if the date of surgery was 15/6/77 then the registrar would write 15/9/77, 15/12/77, 15/3/78, 15/6/78, etc. (giving the dates of follow-up form submission for 2 years) onto the appropriate section of the Confirmation of Registration Form.

8) Lastly, the registrar signs the Confirmation of Registration Form and separates the copies. One copy (the yellow copy) is filed at the operations office, the original (the top copy) is sent to the statistical office, and the bottom copy (the pink copy) is sent to the participant. The date that the copy of the Confirmation Form (Form A) was sent to the institution is entered onto the appropriate line of the Treatment Assignment List.

Once the randomized treatment is given over the phone, it is never to be changed. If the registrar made an error (e. g., choosing the wrong page) the lists are corrected as much as possible at the operations office, entering the patient on the next available correct treatment line, but *under no circumstances* is a randomized treatment assignment to be changed.

Similarly, if the institution calls back with a correction for the stratification factor (or such) the same procedure is followed. The randomization books are corrected as much as possible, but the treatment remains the same.

The patient log is numbered sequentially. As patients are entered on study, a number is assigned from this log. The patient's name (if available), clinic sequence number, and institution are entered here. As subsequent forms are received, the date received is recorded in the log in the appropriate column.

## 4.3 Blank Forms Distribution

Upon initial receipt of forms, the operations office should distribute them to the participating institutions according to anticipated accrual. A few copies of each form should be retained by the operations office to send to institutions whose accrual exceeds expectation.

An initial mailing to each institution should include forms B, C, D, E, and F in proportion 2 : 2 : 2 : 8 : 24 respectively. For example one institution might be sent 20 B Forms, 20 C Forms, 20 D Forms, 80 E Forms, and 240 F Forms.

Included in the initial mailing to each institution should be an updated copy of the protocol and a Forms Submission Timing Sheet.

Form A (Confirmation of Registration Form) and Forms V1 and V2 (Record Review Forms) will not be mailed out to the institutions. Form A is generated from the operations office at the time of patient randomization. Forms V1 and V2 are generated from the statistical center.

All forms used for the study will be prepared by the statistical center. After an initial bulk mailing, the operations office should notify the statistical center of impending shortage of any form (well in advance, if possible). If there is some delay in the availability of forms, photo copies may be used as a temporary measure.

## 4.4 Patient Files

Patient files consist of manila folders for each patient's records. These folders should be ordered by randomization number to match the manner in which the files will be organized at the statistical center. Each folder should be identified with the patient's randomization number, patient's name (or clinic sequence number), and institution. The records within each folder should be kept in chronological order. The use of an "out card" for folders extracted for any reason is recommended.

## 4.5 Reception and Distribution of Forms

As each form is received, it should be stamped (or marked) with the date received, and the corresponding entry made in the patient log. Forms received from the institutions should have two copies remaining (the top white copy and the middle yellow copy), the institution keeping one copy (the bottom pink copy). If the institution did not keep their copy, it should be mailed back. The two copies should be separated, one (the yellow copy) filed at the operations office and the original (the top white copy) mailed to the statistical center. It is suggested that the mailing of forms to the statistical center be made once a week to prevent unknown loss.
Once a patient is randomized the institution is committed to submit forms on that patient. If a nonprotocol treatment was given (inadvertently or precipitated by the patient's condition) it is still necessary for the forms to be submitted so that the case may be evaluated.

## 4.6 Mail Procedure to the Statistical Center

For each mailing, a list of forms should be prepared which gives the patient's study number, type of form, and latest recorded date of form (for follow-up forms and flow sheets only). Each envelope should be numbered (starting with 1) and the number entered on the corresponding list of forms mailed. The date mailed should also be on the list. If more than one envelope is required, separate lists should be prepared for each envelope. The lists of forms included in each mailing should be retained by the operations office in a "mail file."
When mail is received at the statistical center, a record will be kept of the envelope number. If one envelope is missing, a search will be instituted and should the search fail, duplicates of the forms will be requested by envelope number from the operations office. The mail log will then provide the list of forms which can be copied and sent to the statistical center.

## 4.7 Clarification Requests

These requests for data are to be sent to the respective investigators and the responses returned to the operations office.
A copy of the reply to individual letters (and any other material for which the operations office does not have a back-up copy) should be filed in the patient's folder and the original mailed to the statistical center.

## 4.8 Computerized Requests and Study Status Lists

Computerized lists reporting the current clinical status of the patients, the current status of the patients' records, and requests for missing information for each institution should be sent to the operations office by the statistical center. The operations office should separate these lists and forward them to the participating institutions.
The operations office should maintain a copy of the computerized request lists and monitor the response from the institutions, contacting them if necessary. Responses to a computerized listing should consist of forms which are to be processed in the usual fashion.

## 4.9 Records Review

Upon receipt of a Record Review Form (V1 or V2) from the statistical center, the form should be stamped (or marked) with the date received and entered into the patient log. The patient's folder is then to be extracted from the file, the Review Form inserted, and the file given to the study coordinator for review.
When review is completed by the study coordinator, copies of the Review Form should be separated for filing and distribution; one copy (pink copy) to be sent to the institution that entered the patient, one copy (yellow copy) filed in patient's folder, and the original (top white copy) sent to the statistical center. When the final review is completed, the patient's file should be marked "final."

## 4.10 Biostatistical Reports

A copy and the original of each biostatistical report should be sent to the operations office for reproduction and dissemination.

## 4.11 Annual Meetings

The coordinating center organizes annual meetings of project participants to review the progress of the study, treatment administration, complications, and data submissions. In addition, separate meetings of speciality subgroups, e.g., group pathologists, are arranged. While the study is in progress the study group reviews relevant scientific work in order to design upcoming clinical trials before closure of the ongoing trial.

# 5 Statistical Center Specific Activities

## 5.1 Mail Logging and Filing

It is the responsibility of the data manager to review all incoming patient information received at the statistical center and transfer it to a computer file. All data are entered on 3-part NCR forms. The last copy is retained by the investigator, the middle copy is retained at the operations office and the original is sent to the statistical center. When a patient is entered on study, the operations office completes the Confirmation of Registration Form. With the exception of the Case Review Forms, all other data forms originate at the institutions.

Forms are mailed weekly to the statistical center in serially numbered envelopes. A forms log of each envelope's contents is retained at the operations office and a copy is included in each envelope.

When the mail is received, the statistical center data manager should:

1) Check the serial number on the envelope for continuity and file the copy of the forms log received with each envelope.
2) Stamp each piece of mail with the date of arrival.
3) Record the total number of forms received. These totals are given to the data base administrator on a biweekly basis to monitor the data processing activities.
4) Enter each new patient onto the forms log as the Confirmation Forms are received. Receipt of each form is noted in the appropriate column. Refer to Appendix 1.1 for sequence of the forms. An example of the forms log is given in Appendix 9.
5) Maintain a running total of accrual by hospital and treatment in the forms log.

All forms are filed according to study. Within each study, forms are filed according to patient number and type of form.

## 5.2 General Forms Review

### 5.2.1 General Rules

Each form is reviewed for errors, inconsistencies, and missing data. Eligibility and compliance to protocol requirements are checked. Each form is viewed in context with previous forms received.

### 5.2.2 Query Letters

If a form contains errors or inconsistencies or is lacking information, a request for clarification is sent to the investigator, via the operations office. Forms may be photocopied, the missing or questionable area circled, and the form returned with the clarification letter. Questions of eligibility, protocol compliance, or consistently inadequate or incorrect reporting of data are also brought to the attention of the investigator in this manner. Clear-cut violation of eligibility criteria are noted on a comment record and on a V1 record. The investigator should be reminded in the form letter that the patient should be followed though ineligible.

### 5.2.3 Comment Records

Comment Records are literal descriptions of events which become part of the computer file. They are used to:
1) Remind the data manager to check subsequent forms for clarification of questionable items (e.g., the positive paraesophageal nodes on the surgery form must be checked against the histology form to determine eligibility).
2) Alert the statistician to problems such as ineligibility or protocol violations.
3) Expand on a data item which cannot be adequately described in the code provided.
4) Inform the participant of the patient's status. A portion of the comment record is reserved for comments which will appear on patient listings (e.g., ineligibility or protocol violation).

### 5.2.4 Problems

Any medical question which cannot be resolved by communication with the investigator should be referred to the study coordinator. Unusual problems of eligibility and protocol violations should be discussed with the statistician and if necessary, referred to the study coordinator. Any general misinterpretation of the protocol or trend toward undesirable performance by a single institution should be communicated to the statistician and the study coordinator.

## 5.3 Coding Conventions

Two types of variables, categorical and scalar, are recorded by the study forms. Categorical variables are variables whose values are codes assigned to literal or grouped answers, e.g., "1"-No, "2"-Yes. A negative response (the investigator states unknown or unobtainable) should be coded "9". A nonresponse (left blank by investigator but may be necessary) or an illogical response should be coded "8". Scalar variables are actual values such as height, weight, and laboratory values. The actual value should be entered in the space provided. If the value exceeds the alloted space, the highest possible value (e.g., 99 in a two-column field) should be entered. This should be interpreted as a greater value. The actual value is then entered on a comment record. A negative response (the investigator states unknown or unob-tainable) should be coded "−1" (right justified). A nonresponse (left blank by investigator but may be necessary) or illogical response should be coded "−2" (right justified).
Components of a data item may be defined as separate variables, e.g., a date (D, M, Y) is considered to be three variables. An unknown date would be entered as "−1 −1 −1".

## 5.4 Review of Specific Forms

### 5.4.1 Confirmation of Registration Form (Form A)

*Patient's Name.* The spelling should be rechecked when the first form from the institution is received, as names are frequently misspelled.
*Clinic Sequence Number.* If the numbers exceed the allocated space, only the last five digits are entered.
*Eligibility Questions.* All questions should be answered "1" (no). The date of randomization should be within 10 days after date of surgery. If not, the investigator should be contacted for the reason.
*Cancellations.* Cancellations are recorded in column 52, using the following codes:

    "1" – Wrong diagnoses, not cancer,
    "2" – primary other than lung.

### 5.4.2 Clinical and Preoperative Form (Form B)

*Q.1.* The year of birth must be $\leq 70$ years prior to study entry.
*Q.6.* If the weight loss is $> 10$ kg the bone marrow biopsy (Q.20) should have been performed.
*Q.7–Q.13.* Answers must be "1" or the patient is ineligible.
*Q.9.* Chronic disease should not be anything listed in Appendix 1.2.
*Q.14–Q.17.* One of these tests should be performed if there is clinical suspicion of liver involvement.
*Q.19.* If this question concerning mediastinoscopy is answered "3" or "5", the patient is ineligible.
*Q.20.* See Q.6.
*Q.21–Q.30.* If there are any distant metastases, the patient is ineligible.
*Q.30–Q.34.* $T > 2, N > 1, M > 0$, or disease stage $> 2$ indicate ineligibility. If any of these parameters are exceeded, the histology form should be checked for confirmation.

### 5.4.3 Surgery Form (Form C)

*Q.1.* The date of resection and (Q.2) type of resection should be consistent with the Confirmation Form.
*Q.13.* If other nodes are involved compare with the Histology Form.
*Q.14.* If answered "1", the Histology Form should be checked for confirmation. (This question is sometimes answered incorrectly simply because it requires changing to a code "2" for no immediately following a list of "1"-no answers.)
*Q.15.* The location of the primary should be consistent with Q.2.
*Q.16.* If the tumor size is $> 3$ cm, the T classification on Histology Form should be "2".

### 5.4.4 Histology and Study Treatment Form (Form D)

*Q.2–Q.4, Q.8, Q.10.* If answered "2", the patient is ineligible.
*Q.11, Q.12.* If answered "2", the "Ineligibility-specific" section of the protocol should be reviewed for eligibility criteria.

*Q.14.* If answered "2", the patient is ineligible.

*Q.19.* The histologic classification should be squamous, adenocarcinoma, or large cell.

*Q.20.* The randomized therapy should be consistent with the Confirmation Form.

*Q.21.* The date of administration should be between days 6 and 10 postoperatively.

Any clear case of ineligibility should be recorded on the Eligibility Review Form (Form V1).

### 5.4.5 Follow-up Form (Form E)

*Q.1 and Q.2.* The "Records to be kept" section of the protocol gives the submission schedule.

Any lengthy gap between follow-ups should be questioned. Minor gaps are to be adjusted by changing the initial date (i.e., by a few days). The sequence number should be entered in columns 13−14 of the heading, beginning with 01. The sequence is by due date, e.g., month 3 = 01, month 6 = 02. A dummy E1 record consisting of the first 15 columns of the computer record and the date the follow-up was due in columns 24−29 (date the follow-up ended) should be entered under the following conditions:

1) There are no gaps in the dates between previous forms and the current forms.
2) The date ended is not ± 45 days from actual due date.

*Q.4−Q.7.* If Q. 3 is other than "1", an event should be specified. The site should be entered on a comment record.

*Q.8−Q.11.* If answered "2", details should be entered on a comment record.

*Q.12−Q.19.* These questions should be blank unless the patient is dead or lost to follow-up. If lost to follow-up, the reason should be entered on a comment record.

### 5.4.6 Flow Sheet Form (Form F)

Only one column will be completed on each form. The date of visit should be checked for time sequence. Sequence in columns 13−14 of the heading should be entered as follows:

|            | Time point                       | Sequence no.     |
| ---------- | -------------------------------- | ---------------- |
| 1st column | Presurgery                       | 01               |
| 2nd column | Before *C. parvum* or placebo    | 02               |
| 3rd column | After *C. parvum* or placebo     | 03               |
| 4th column | All subsequent visits            | 04, 3 months     |
|            |                                  | 05, 6 months, etc. |

All sequencing is by the date the form is scheduled. If the investigator states that no information is available for any of the first three timepoints, a "1" should be entered in column 16 of the computer record (an additional box in the heading) to indicate a dummy form. This method is not used for subsequent follow-ups. Once informed that a flow sheet for a subsequent time period (3 months, 6 months, etc.) is not forthcoming, an F1 record containing the first 15 columns of the computer record and the scheduled date of visit in columns 18–23 is entered.

*Q.2–Q.10, Q.23.* A "–2" (right justified) is used to indicate no answers. The investigator will use "–1" to indicate not done or not available.

*Q.11–Q.15.* If the liver enzymes are abnormal before surgery (column 1), the B form should be checked to determine if at least one required test was performed.

*Q.16–Q.22.* These questions should not be left blank (The code "0" is provided for no complications or reactions).

*5.4.7 Eligibility Review Forms (Forms V1 and V2)*

Upon receipt of sufficient information to identify a clear-cut case of ineligibility a V1 Form is prepared and mailed to the operations office for review by the study coordinator. As soon as the B, C, and D Forms have been received for each patient, the V1 Form is routinely prepared and mailed. Upon receipt of a report of a first recurrence or metastases a V2 Form is prepared and handled in the same manner as the V1 Form. The V2 Form is prepared once more when the patient has died and the case is ready for closing. A final version of the V2 form is not yet available.

All case review forms originate with the data manager at the statistical center, where they are entered on the computer. A copy is retained while the form is sent to the study coordinator for review and a decision on questionable cases. The study coordinator sends a copy to the investigator and returns the original to the statistical center. The original is reprocessed, making any necessary changes on the computer.

These case review forms serve as:
1) An administrative record of protocol adherence and data quality;
2) a tool for analysis by identifying eligibility and evaluability;
3) a method of establishing consistent interpretations of data;
4) a means of resolving disagreements with the study coordinator, investigator, data manager, and statistician;
5) a flag that a case has been closed.

## 5.5 File Organization

As files are processed, data are entered on computer files. Patient records are retained as paper files to document computerized data. Computer back-up files are maintained in the event of a system breakdown. Computer files are stored on magnetic disks. The data for each study is maintained on a separate computer file. The data is on-line at all times, i.e., it can be retrieved without mounting tapes or requiring any other operator intervention. In addition, this means the data can be viewed and interrogated through terminals.

The data records within each study are ordered by patient number, type of form, and chronological sequence of that form. Each record consists of 80 columns and is uniquely identified in the first 15 columns.

To simplify data retrieval, auxiliary files have been created which describe the variables on the data records. Each data item or variable has a unique four-character identification "key" in the variable description file (VDF). This file is also referred to as the Data Dictionary.

The main uses of the VDF are:
1) To describe the format of each study file;
2) to aid in retrieving information (the VDF can be used with other computer programs to search out any data on the computer file);
3) to allow the update program to identify out of range values.


## 5.6 File Maintenance

Once reviewed, the forms are batched by type of form and given to the data entry operator. Data entry is accomplished either through keypunched cards or entry on a Datapoint terminal.


### 5.6.1 Keypunch

Data is recorded on 80 column IBM cards which are verified for operator accuracy. Forms and cards are returned to the data manager who then has the cards read into the computer. The keypunch method is only used as a backup system.


### 5.6.2 Datapoint

Data is entered on a disk in the same format as the keypunched cards. Range values are checked by a computer program using the VDF. Forms are returned to the data manager. The data is transmitted and the appropriate program is initiated by the Datapoint operator.


### 5.6.3 Update Program

Data for each protocol is updated by first submitting an update file for execution by the main program, checking the update listing for error messages, correcting the errors found, and then merging the cleaned new data into the protocol data file.


## 5.7 Data Retrieval

Data is retrieved from the protocol data file by the basic statistical center retrieval program. This program only requires specification of the appropriate data "keys" in the variable description file. The extracted data is then ready for analysis with the standard statistical center analysis programs.


## 5.8 Computer Listings

From the data files it is possible to obtain various types of listings. A sample listing of the data file may be found in Appendix 8.

### 5.8.1 Patient Listings

Patient listings are generated periodically for each institution. They contain the patient's name, study case number, clinic sequence number, treatment assignment, date entered, date of disease recurrence, date of last contact or death, plus remarks concerning cancellations, ineligibility, or protocol violations. This gives the institution a complete listing of patients entered on the study and informs them of the status of computer files for each patient. A sample listing may be found in Appendix 4.

### 5.8.2 Data Request

A request for overdue forms is generated periodically and sent to the operations office for distribution to the institutions. An example may be found in Appendix 3.

## 5.9 Manuals

In anticipation of an increasing use of data managers (identified as data handlers in some European institutions), a data management manual has been prepared.

## 5.10 Workshops

Workshops will be held as the need arises. The workshops stress:
1) The vital role of the data manager in the collection of study data;
2) the necessity for smooth and effcient communication between the data manager at the institution and the statistical center;
3) the need for accurate, complete, and prompt reporting of data.

Past experience has demonstrated the beneficial aspects of the workshop in providing a forum for the exchange of ideas and problem solving. The first workshop was held three months after the trial started.

## *Appendix 1. Protocol*

### Project Title

Locoregional and systemic immunostimulation as adjuvant therapy in radical resected bronchogenic squamous cell carcinoma, adenocarcinoma and large cell carcinoma.

### Patient Population

Patients with histologically proven squamous cell carcinoma, adenocarcinoma or large cell carcinoma and classified post surgically as $T_1N_0M_0$, $T_2N_0M_0$, $T_1N_1M_0$, or $T_2N_1M_0$.

### Patient Entry

Patients will be entered (randomized) into the study after surgery but before the 10th day postoperatively.

### Schema

(Stratify by type of surgery)

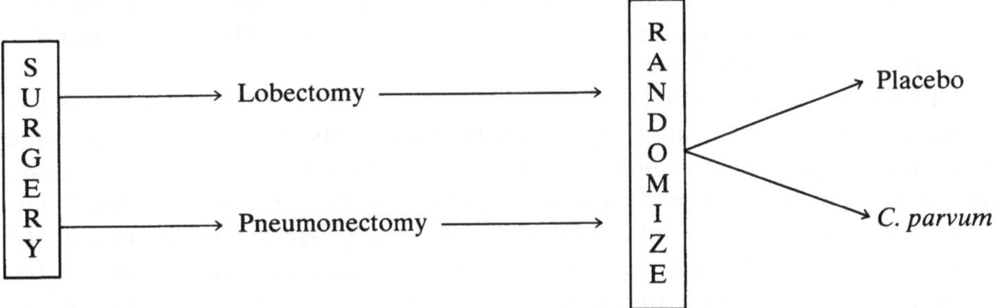


### *C. parvum*

7 mg intrapleurally once between day 6 and 10 postoperatively.

### Study Activated

July 1, 1977.

### For Randomization

Call the Study Operations. Office.

June 1977
Revised December 1977

**Objectives**

1) The study aims to determine if locoregional immunostimulation by intrapleural *C. parvum* in patients with "radical resected bronchogenic non-oat cell carcinoma can
   a) increase the tumor recurrence-free interval;
   b) increase survival;
   c) change general immune status and tumor associated immune responses.
2) The study aims to identify high risk patients within operable bronchogenic non-oat cell carcinoma after biologic and immunomorphological studies.


**Project Background**

Bronchogenic carcinoma is one of the most common tumors and the frequency is still increasing in many countries. The overall prognosis of patients with bronchogenic carcinoma is poor. The 5-year survival including all stages varies between 5% and 15%.

For curative therapy, surgical resection remains the most important therapy. Even after so-called radical resection, the results are difficult to accept. Two-thirds to three-quarters of these patients will die because of locoregional and/or distant tumor recurrence within the first 5 years postoperatively. Intrathoracic recurrence occurs in more than 50%. In spite of so-called radical removal of the tumor, there is in reality a high number of patients with locoregional incomplete resection and/or invisible microdissemination at time of surgery. Search for a nonsurgical adjuvant therapy which may be active both locoregionally and systemically is therefore motivated. Postoperative radiotherapy has not improved survival in operable cases, nor has chemotherapy so far fulfilled the hopes.

The role of immunotherapy in itself or as an adjuvant treatment modality remains to be investigated. Findings indicate that a direct relation exists between histologic signs of host immune reactions in regional lymph nodes and prognosis in bronchogenic squamous cell carcinoma. These observations are consistent with other indirect data showing a relationship between immunocompetence and prognosis in lung cancer [6]. A decrease in the ability to react immunologically with increasing tumor burden has been noticed in patients with pulmonary cancer [4, 9, 17]. Other investigations produced indirect evidence indicating that a nonspecific enhancement of host immune responsiveness in patients with pulmonary tumors may be correlated with improved prognosis. Various studies on human cancer patients, both nonrandomized and controlled, support the notion of a beneficial effect of immunostimulation [14], with materials such as BCG [8, 13, 16, 22], *C. parvum* [6], tumor extract, or antigenically modified, reinjected tumor cells [1, 22]. Cross-transfused leukocytes have also been reported to improve the lung cancer patient's defense mechanisms [5]. In the same vein, the occurrence of postoperative empyema in such cases seems to stimulate the host's reactivity towards the neoplastic press [14]. Recent data from a randomized clinical controlled study indicate a significant delay of tumor recurrence of operable bronchogenic carcinoma after postoperative administration of intrapleural BCG. Totally, however, only 39 Stage I patients were included [13].

The present study aims to investigate the role of combined local and systemic administration of *C. parvum* after "radical resection of bronchogenic squamous cell carcinoma ($T_{1/2}$, $N_{0/1}$, $M_0$). The high number of patients with bronchogenic carcinoma, the early tumor recurrence after "radical" resection (minimal tumor burden — realistic for immunotherapy) and the inefficiency of present treatment modalities offers a realistic opportunity to analyze conclusively and in a short time whether the proposed immunotherapy could improve prognosis.

## Patient Selection

### Patient Eligibility

All patients with histologically proven squamous cell carcinoma, adenocarcinoma, or large cell carcinoma and *classified postsurgically* as:
$T_1N_0M_0$
$T_2N_0M_0$
$T_1N_1M_0$
$T_2N_1M_0$
will be considered for this trial.

### Patient Ineligibility — General

Patients will not be considered for this trial if they:
1) Are over 70 years of age;
2) Have had any previous malignancy [except skin cancer (basal cell)];
3) Have had previous treatment by irradiation, cytotoxic drugs, or immunosuppressants (e.g., steroids);
4) Are geographically unsuitable;
5) Are medically unsuitable (see Appendix 1.2).

### Patient Ineligibility — Specific

Patients will not be considered for this trial if they have:
1) Positive mediastinoscopy; for example, metastasis in lymph nodes of the ipsi- and/or contralateral tracheobronchial angle and/or the tracheal bifurcation (subcarinal).
2) Evidence for tumor spread in the contralateral lung and/or for distant metastases.
3) Had operations other than standard resections.
4) Histologic evidence of neoplastic growth at the bronchial resection line.
5) Tumors not confined to the lung; that is to say tumors which have extended outside the pleura visceralis.
6) Tumors of the main bronchus closer than 2 cm to the tracheal carina.
7) Cytologically positive pleural exudate.
8) Histologically proven metastases in mediastinal, subaortic, or paraesophageal lymph nodes (operation specimen).
9) Paralysis of phrenic and/or recurrence nerve of any cause.

**Stratification and Randomization**

Patients will be entered into the study after surgery but before the 10th day postoperatively. Each participating institute/clinic agrees to enter into the randomized trial *all* eligible patients.

Tumor size ($T_1/T_2$) and localization are important for prognosis and are partly reflected in the type of operation done (lobectomy or pneumonectomy). To balance the groups with respect to prognosis within each participating clinic, the patients are divided (stratified) into two groups, depending on whether lobectomy or pneumonectomy has been done. Within each stratification group the patients will be assigned to a randomized treatment regimen − surgery plus placebo or surgery plus immunotherapy.

After a patient has been found to meet all the eligibility requirements of the study, patient randomization will take place by telephoning the study operations office in Bern. The investigator should be prepared to supply the following information:

1) Clinic's name,
2) Patient's name (optional),
3) The clinic sequence number (an institution identification number assigned to that patient),
4) Patient's age,
5) Whether the patient has had any previous malignancy,
6) Whether the patient has been previously treated by irradiation, cytotoxic drugs, or immunosuppressants,
7) Whether there are any contraindications to *C. parvum,*
8) Date of surgery,
9) Type of operation (lobectomy or pneumonectomy).

The treatment to be given that patient − surgery plus placebo or surgery plus *C. parvum* − and a study number (also known as randomization number) will be assigned by the operations office before the telephone call is terminated. This study number will be used on all future correspondence for that patient. After the telephone call, the operations office will also send a form to the clinic confirming the assigned treatment and study number.


**Surgery**

The details of surgery will be specified on the study forms. Some regional, tumor-free lymph nodes are to be dissected out separately and cut by the pathologist for later immunomorphological studies.


**Treatment Administration**

*General: Applies to All Patients*

*Insertion of Catheter.* At the time of operation a catheter is placed at the tracheal bifurcation, at the site of the bronchial resection line. This position of the catheter is fixed by a catgut suture.

*Time of Injection. C. parvum* or placebo should be administered between day 6 and 10 postoperatively, and after removal of the thoracic draining tubes.

*Use of Antibiotics.* The administration of antibiotics postoperatively will be done according to each clinic's tradition.

## Immunotherapy

*Choice of the Intrapleural Route.* The rationale for using the intrapleural route of administration for tumors of the bronchus is that, in animal experimental systems, the strongest immunotherapeutic effects with both *C. parvum* and BCG have been observed when they are injected into, or in the vicinity of, the tumor. The intrapleural route is therefore an attempt to bring the *C. parvum* in proximity to the tumor cells.

Intrapleural injection of BCG in rats has been shown to have a therapeutic effect on intrapleurally injected tumor cells [17]. The first results of a clinical trial of immunotherapy of lung cancer with intrapleural BCG have recently appeared [13]. A single injection of $10^7$ viable units of BCG was given after surgery (usually 3−5 days afterwards). At the time of the report, 24 months after the beginning of the trial, 9 of the 22 control Stage I patients had developed recurrences and 5 had died. There were no recurrences or deaths among the 17 BCG-treated Stage I patients ($p = 0.003$). The BCG treatment was without effect in patients with more advanced disease. Clinical experience with *C. parvum* injected subcutaneously or intravenously has shown that doses in this range are tolerated [3, 6].

A Phase I pilot study has, therefore, been undertaken within the trial to determine the side effects that follow intrapleural injection [11].

In the mouse a dose of 5−50 μg is effective both for therapy of tumors by injection of *C. parvum* directly into the tumor [19] or for stimulating the immune response to tumor antigens by injecting mixtures of *C. parvum* and irradiated tumor cells [2, 20]. The appropriate human equivalent doses are 0.7−7 mg/M$^2$.

## Choice of *C. parvum* Rather than BCG

The mechanisms of the antitumor effects of *C. parvum* and BCG are probably very similar. They both activate macrophages, and also stimulate the host immune response to tumor antigens. *C. parvum* possesses three advantages over BCG:

a) It is used as a killed bacterial suspension, whereas BCG is living. In the clinical trial of McKneally et al. [13], all patients were treated with isoniazid to prevent overgrowth of bacilli, a known danger of BCG injection.

b) The activity of *C. parvum* is very stable. If the *C. parvum* is kept at 4° C there is little loss of activity after 1−2 years. The BCG preparations are less suitable.

c) The antitumor activity of *C. parvum* in animal experimental systems has been found to be stronger than that of BCG when direct comparisons are made [10, 21].

*Administration of C. parvum*

One ampoule of 7 mg *C. parvum* diluted in 10 cc sterile physiologic sodium chloride is injected slowly through the catheter. While doing this, draw up the catheter slowly (approximately 5 cm) so that the *C. parvum* is distributed over a larger area. The catheter is rinsed with 5 cc sterile sodium chloride thereafter.
Additional care should be taken if *C. parvum* is administered to patients with coexisting disorders in which there is evidence of abnormal immune function, i.e., collagen disease, or patients receiving regular barbiturate therapy.

*Treatment Monitoring.* Patient's temperature, pulse, respiration and blood pressure should be recorded hourly during *C. parvum* infusion and 4-hourly for 48 h after completion of the infusion.

*Dose of Intrapleural C. parvum.* The choice of the 7 mg dose of *C. parvum* was based on the results of the pilot study [11].

*Administration of Placebo*

For patients randomized to receive surgery plus placebo, as a placebo 10 cc sterile physiologic sodium chloride is injected slowly through the catheter, in the same fashion as the administration of *C. parvum*.

**Study Parameters for Patient Follow-up**

These are shown on Table 1. All information is recorded on the study forms.
The following points should be noted:
1) The aim of the follow-up is to determine the time of tumor recurrence, possible changes in the immunoprofile of the patient and survival.
2) To answer the question of recurrence-free interval, it is mandatory that follow-up is done regularly and carefully.
3) The patient will be followed up in each clinic every 3rd month during the first 3 years postoperatively and every 6 months thereafter. A follow-up form [Form E] is filled in each time and sent to the operations office. Each time the patient is examined at the institution (every 3rd month or more frequently) a flow sheet [Form F] is also prepared. The day of operation, to which control times are related, is considered Day 0.
4) The high frequency of tumor recurrence within the first 2−3 years makes it realistic to evaluate in a rather short time whether an effect of added immunotherapy occurs. Study results and closure of trial will be discussed among the participants at the annual meeting 1 and 2 years after the start of the trial.
5) Evaluation of the effect of immunotherapy will be made by comparison of the randomization groups with respect to three criteria:
   a) The duration of the initial *disease-free interval,* measured from the date of surgery;

**Table 1.** Study parameters

| Parameters | Prior to surgical procedures (within 1 week) | Before *C. parvum* or placebo (within 24 h) | After *C. parvum* or placebo (between 24–48 h) | Every 3 months |
|---|---|---|---|---|
| History and physical exam. | × | | | |
| Clinical exam. | × | | | × |
| Lung X-ray (P.A. and lateral) | × | | | × |
| Performance status | × | | | × |
| Blood differential and hematologic studies [neutrophils (seg), neutrophils (unseg), eosinophils, basophils, lymphocytes, monocytes, WBC, platelets, and erythrocyte sedimentation rate] | ×[a] | × | × | ×[e] |
| Liver enzymes (SGOT, SGPT, alkaline phosphatase, LAP, and $\gamma$-GT) | × | | | × |
| Laparoscopy [b] | | | | |
| Liver scintiscan [b] | | | | |
| (Mini) laparotomy [b] | | | | |
| Ultrasound [c] | | | | |
| Pulmonary function tests [c] | | | | |
| Mediastinoscopy [f] | | | | |
| Bone marrow biopsy [d] | | | | |

[a] Blood differential before *any* surgical procedures and (facultative) a blood sample ($2 \times 10$ ml), from which serum is separated, frozen ($-20°$ C) and stored (serum bank)

[b] Laparoscopy and/or liver scintiscan and/or minilaparotomy is done routinely only when serum enzyme and/or clinical appearance is suspect for liver metastasis

[c] Optional

[d] Bone marrow biopsy has to be done in cases of more than 10 kg weight loss within 6 months (facultative)

[e] Serum sample to be stored from serum bank ($2 \times 10$ ml) (facultative)

[f] Mandatory if peripheral lesion

    b) The distribution of patients relapsing in specified time intervals after surgery according to the type of relapse (local, regional, and/or distant tumor recurrence);

    c) The *duration of survival,* measured from the date of surgery.

6) If symptoms of local and/or distant tumor recurrence are found, the patient is investigated further, to establish possible tumor growth.

7) The patient should be assessed by a colleague identified in the trial protocol.

8) There will be histometric analysis of regional lymph nodes for an immunomorphology study and evaluation of cellular infiltrates within or in the neighborhood of the primary tumor. Immunomorphological changes will be analyzed and correlated with histology of the primary tumor and clinical development.

9) Depending on the capacity within the different institutes participating, tumor associated immune response and general immune parameters changing with immunotherapy (facultative) will be investigated after further discussion. A horizontal follow-up of all individual patients allocated to the study of these parameters is not judged possible.

10) Autopsy should be carried out whenever possible. This is very important and a specific form will be prepared by the participating pathologists. A number of patients will continue to remain disease free for the duration of the trial.

**Patient Management**

After evidence of relapse from local recurrence or distant metastasis, patients may be treated for their disease according to local practice. The follow-up of such a patient is continued to the ultimate end point, survival. It is recognized that observation with respect to one or both of these end points may be terminated by death from unrelated causes or by losing contact with the patient altogether. Once randomized, all patients must be followed-up, even though they may later be found ineligible, e.g., histology may arrive later which would make the patient ineligible.

**Pathology**

All specimens will be examined and diagnosed by the pathologist of the center concerned. The material will be classified according to the current WHO Histologic Classification and the diagnosis reported on the study forms. For the sake of uniformity, there will be a central review of the material, involving a reference pathologist.

For each patient the following material will be submitted to the operations office:

1) The original slide used for diagnosis (when possible),

2) At least two unstained sections,

3) The site(s) and preparation technique of the diagnostic material.

The material should be permanently identified by patient name (or clinic sequence number), institution, and patient study number. The recommended technique for routine work-up of surgical or autopsy specimen(s) is:

1) Fixation of specimen: aqueous solution or formaldehyde 4%, isotonic, neutral;

2) Embedding: paraffin or paraplast blocks;

3) Staining: H & E routine stains, possibly others;
4) Mounting: routine mounting on micro slides (76 × 26 mm, 0.8−1.0 mm thickness, white, precleaned); covering with microscopic glass cover slips (24 × 40 mm or 24 × 50 mm);
5) Type of tissue to be worked up:
   a) Primary tumor (if not resected before) including its border,
   b) Bronchial resection rim,
   c) Regional lymph nodes, some with metastasis *and* some without metastasis,
   d) Peripheral lung tissue plus pleural surface where inflammatory changes due to *C. parvum* are suspected.

## Statistical Considerations

In order to balance the treatment groups with respect to prognosis, the patients will be stratified according to type of surgery (lobectomy or pneumonectomy). Within each stratification group the patients will be assigned to a randomized treatment regimen (surgery plus placebo or surgery plus *C. parvum*) using the procedure given in the section entitled "Stratification and Randomization".

It is anticipated that 400 patients (200 per treatment arm) entered in 1 year and followed for 3 years will be required for this study. If the disease-free interval is in fact increased by 50% (i.e., a change from 3 years to 4.5 years), this increase will be detected with a probability of 86% using a statistical test with $p = 0.05$.

Frequent review of study results will make it possible to terminate this study at an earlier date if it is determined that continued follow-up is unlikely to alter the study findings.

## Records to Be Kept

The keeping of accurate and consistent records is essential to a cooperative study. The following forms are to be submitted at the indicated times by the participating institution for each patient:

| Form | To be submitted |
| --- | --- |
| Form B − Clinical and preoperative form | Within 1 week prior to surgery |
| Form C − Surgery form | After surgery |
| Form D − Histology and study treatment form | After administration of *C. parvum* or placebo |
| Form E − Follow-up form | Every 3 months after surgery for first 3 years, and every 6 months thereafter |
| Form F − Flow sheet | Prior to surgery (within 1 week), before *C. parvum* or placebo (within 24 h), after *C. parvum* or placebo (between 24 and 48 h) and each time the patient is examined thereafter |

Additional forms may be added for specific investigations.

The time of submission of each form is presented in a sequential fashion in the "Forms Submission Timing Sheet" given in Appendix 1.1.

All forms should be completed and mailed at the time indicated. The flow sheets (Form F) should accompany the corresponding follow-up form (Form E), which is to be submitted every 3 months for the first 3 years, and every 6 months thereafter. After completion of the forms, the bottom (pink) copy should be removed and kept on file at the institution. The two remaining copies (the top white copy and the middle yellow copy) should be sent to the operations office.

## Informed Consent

It is important that the Helsinki (WHO) recommendations are fulfilled. It is recommended that before patients enter the trial, there should be informed consent. However, due to local variations and patient–doctor relationships the way of doing this has to be left to the discretion of each center.

## Policy

1) Data from all patients will be summarized twice a year and the result will be communicated to all the participants. There will be a yearly meeting between the participants.
2) Similarly, details of any pathologic or clinical features which correlate with improved or impaired results in treatment will be circulated to those taking part.
3) When publishing results from the trial, every participant and center involved is to be included.
4) Every participant should be free to communicate the results orally, preferably under the mutual trial name. Twenty copies of abstracts, etc. should be sent to the coordinating center for registration and distribution among participants.
5) The trial is a true cooperative study, working according to the principle of "one for all and all for one". No one person should be identified more than anyone else. When special investigations are needed from outside experts, they can be invited and identified as guest workers.
6) When joining and cementing a collaborative trial, the individual participating member should try to canalize collaboration with other possible study groups through our trial group, not only regarding the ongoing study, but also in the logical development of the trial, which will be decided within the group.

## Appendix 1.1. Forms Submission Timing Sheet

Forms to be submitted by the participating institution for each patient:

| Point in time | Forms to be submitted |
| --- | --- |
| Initial entry | ←Flow sheet (Form F, first column only) within 1 week prior to surgery. Clinical and Preoperative Form (Form B) |
| Surgery | ←Surgery Form (Form C) |
|  | ←Flow sheet (Form F, second column only) within 24 h prior to administration of *C. parvum* or placebo |
| *C. parvum* or placebo | ←Flow sheet (Form F, third column only) between 24–48 h after administration of *C. parvum* or placebo<br>Histology and Study Treatment Form (Form D) |
| 3rd month after surgery | ←Follow-up Form (Form E) (for period of surgery to 3 months), and Flow Sheets for each visit in that period (Form F, column 4 only) |
| 6th month after surgery | ←Follow-up Form (Form E) (for period 3–6 months), and Flow Sheets for each visit in that period (Form F, column 4 only) |
| 3-month periods for the first 3 years and 6-month periods thereafter (First recurrence of disease will take place in one of these periods) | ←Follow-up Forms (Form E) (for 3 month periods for the first 3 years and 6 month periods thereafter) and corresponding Flow Sheets (Form F, column 4 only) |
| Death | ∠Death Form (Form Z)<br>Follow-up Form (Form E) (for last period to death). |

## Appendix 1.2. Contraindications for Administration of *C. parvum*

1) Patients with any severe allergic disorder or history of endotoxic shock.
2) Significant hypertension (i.e., resting diastolic BP > 100 mm Hg), history or signs of ischaemic or valvular heart disease.
3) Current pregnancy.
4) Patients with disturbance of blood clotting mechanisms.
5) Gross impairment of liver or renal function.
6) Long term steroid administration.
7) Primary or secondary cerebral neoplasms.
8) Patients with known thiomersal sensitivity.
9) Coexisting untreated infection.

# Appendix 1.3. Tables for Determination of Surface Area ($m^2$) as a Function of Height (cm) and Weight (kg)



| Height (cm) | Weight (kg) | | | | | | | | | | | | | | | | | | | | | | | | | | | | |
|---|---|---|---|---|---|---|---|---|---|---|---|---|---|---|---|---|---|---|---|---|---|---|---|---|---|---|---|---|---|
| | 4 | 6 | 8 | 10 | 12 | 14 | 16 | 18 | 20 | 22 | 24 | 26 | 28 | 30 | 32 | 34 | 36 | 38 | 40 | 44 | 48 | 52 | 56 | 60 | | | | | |
| 50 | 0.25 | 0.31 | 0.36 | 0.40 | 0.44 | 0.48 | 0.51 | 0.54 | 0.57 | 0.60 | 0.63 | 0.66 | 0.68 | 0.71 | 0.73 | 0.75 | 0.78 | 0.80 | 0.82 | 0.86 | 0.90 | 0.94 | 0.97 | 1.01 | | | | | |
| 55 | 0.26 | 0.32 | 0.37 | 0.42 | 0.46 | 0.50 | 0.53 | 0.57 | 0.60 | 0.63 | 0.66 | 0.68 | 0.71 | 0.74 | 0.76 | 0.78 | 0.81 | 0.83 | 0.85 | 0.90 | 0.94 | 0.98 | 1.01 | 1.05 | | | | | |
| 60 | 0.27 | 0.33 | 0.39 | 0.43 | 0.48 | 0.52 | 0.55 | 0.59 | 0.62 | 0.65 | 0.68 | 0.71 | 0.74 | 0.76 | 0.79 | 0.81 | 0.84 | 0.86 | 0.88 | 0.93 | 0.97 | 1.01 | 1.05 | 1.09 | | | | | |
| 65 | 0.28 | 0.34 | 0.40 | 0.45 | 0.49 | 0.53 | 0.57 | 0.61 | 0.64 | 0.67 | 0.70 | 0.73 | 0.76 | 0.79 | 0.82 | 0.84 | 0.87 | 0.89 | 0.91 | 0.96 | 1.00 | 1.05 | 1.09 | 1.13 | | | | | |
| 70 | 0.29 | 0.36 | 0.41 | 0.46 | 0.51 | 0.55 | 0.59 | 0.63 | 0.66 | 0.69 | 0.73 | 0.76 | 0.79 | 0.81 | 0.84 | 0.87 | 0.89 | 0.92 | 0.94 | 0.99 | 1.04 | 1.08 | 1.12 | 1.16 | | | | | |
| 75 | 0.30 | 0.37 | 0.42 | 0.48 | 0.52 | 0.57 | 0.61 | 0.64 | 0.68 | 0.71 | 0.75 | 0.78 | 0.81 | 0.84 | 0.87 | 0.89 | 0.92 | 0.95 | 0.97 | 1.02 | 1.07 | 1.11 | 1.16 | 1.20 | | | | | |
| 80 | 0.31 | 0.38 | 0.44 | 0.49 | 0.54 | 0.58 | 0.62 | 0.66 | 0.70 | 0.73 | 0.77 | 0.80 | 0.83 | 0.86 | 0.89 | 0.92 | 0.95 | 0.97 | 1.00 | 1.05 | 1.10 | 1.14 | 1.19 | 1.23 | | | | | |
| 85 | 0.31 | 0.39 | 0.45 | 0.50 | 0.55 | 0.60 | 0.64 | 0.68 | 0.72 | 0.75 | 0.79 | 0.82 | 0.85 | 0.88 | 0.91 | 0.94 | 0.97 | 1.00 | 1.02 | 1.08 | 1.13 | 1.17 | 1.22 | 1.26 | | | | | |
| 90 | 0.32 | 0.40 | 0.46 | 0.51 | 0.56 | 0.61 | 0.65 | 0.70 | 0.73 | 0.77 | 0.81 | 0.84 | 0.87 | 0.91 | 0.94 | 0.97 | 0.99 | 1.02 | 1.05 | 1.10 | 1.15 | 1.20 | 1.25 | 1.29 | | | | | |
| 95 | 0.33 | 0.40 | 0.47 | 0.53 | 0.58 | 0.63 | 0.67 | 0.71 | 0.75 | 0.79 | 0.83 | 0.86 | 0.89 | 0.93 | 0.96 | 0.99 | 1.02 | 1.05 | 1.07 | 1.13 | 1.18 | 1.23 | 1.28 | 1.32 | | | | | |

| Height (cm) | Weight (kg) | | | | | | | | | | | | | | | | | | | | | | | | | | | | |
|---|---|---|---|---|---|---|---|---|---|---|---|---|---|---|---|---|---|---|---|---|---|---|---|---|---|---|---|---|---|
| | 12 | 14 | 16 | 18 | 20 | 22 | 24 | 26 | 28 | 30 | 32 | 34 | 36 | 38 | 40 | 42 | 44 | 48 | 52 | 56 | 60 | 64 | 68 | 72 | | | | | |
| 100 | 0.59 | 0.64 | 0.68 | 0.73 | 0.77 | 0.81 | 0.84 | 0.88 | 0.91 | 0.95 | 0.98 | 1.01 | 1.04 | 1.07 | 1.10 | 1.13 | 1.15 | 1.21 | 1.26 | 1.30 | 1.35 | 1.40 | 1.44 | 1.48 | | | | | |
| 105 | 0.60 | 0.65 | 0.70 | 0.74 | 0.78 | 0.82 | 0.86 | 0.90 | 0.93 | 0.97 | 1.00 | 1.03 | 1.06 | 1.09 | 1.12 | 1.15 | 1.18 | 1.23 | 1.28 | 1.33 | 1.38 | 1.43 | 1.47 | 1.52 | | | | | |
| 110 | 0.61 | 0.67 | 0.71 | 0.76 | 0.80 | 0.84 | 0.88 | 0.92 | 0.95 | 0.99 | 1.02 | 1.05 | 1.08 | 1.11 | 1.14 | 1.17 | 1.20 | 1.25 | 1.31 | 1.36 | 1.41 | 1.45 | 1.50 | 1.55 | | | | | |
| 115 | 0.63 | 0.68 | 0.73 | 0.77 | 0.81 | 0.86 | 0.89 | 0.93 | 0.97 | 1.00 | 1.04 | 1.07 | 1.10 | 1.13 | 1.16 | 1.19 | 1.22 | 1.28 | 1.33 | 1.38 | 1.43 | 1.48 | 1.53 | 1.58 | | | | | |
| 120 | 0.64 | 0.69 | 0.74 | 0.79 | 0.83 | 0.87 | 0.91 | 0.95 | 0.99 | 1.02 | 1.06 | 1.09 | 1.12 | 1.15 | 1.19 | 1.22 | 1.24 | 1.30 | 1.36 | 1.41 | 1.46 | 1.51 | 1.56 | 1.60 | | | | | |
| 125 | 0.65 | 0.70 | 0.75 | 0.80 | 0.84 | 0.89 | 0.93 | 0.97 | 1.00 | 1.04 | 1.07 | 1.11 | 1.14 | 1.17 | 1.21 | 1.24 | 1.27 | 1.32 | 1.38 | 1.43 | 1.49 | 1.54 | 1.58 | 1.63 | | | | | |
| 130 | 0.66 | 0.71 | 0.77 | 0.81 | 0.86 | 0.90 | 0.94 | 0.98 | 1.02 | 1.06 | 1.09 | 1.13 | 1.16 | 1.19 | 1.23 | 1.26 | 1.29 | 1.35 | 1.40 | 1.46 | 1.51 | 1.56 | 1.61 | 1.66 | | | | | |
| 135 | 0.67 | 0.73 | 0.78 | 0.83 | 0.87 | 0.92 | 0.96 | 1.00 | 1.04 | 1.07 | 1.11 | 1.15 | 1.18 | 1.21 | 1.25 | 1.28 | 1.31 | 1.37 | 1.43 | 1.48 | 1.53 | 1.59 | 1.64 | 1.69 | | | | | |
| 140 | 0.68 | 0.74 | 0.79 | 0.84 | 0.89 | 0.93 | 0.97 | 1.01 | 1.05 | 1.09 | 1.13 | 1.16 | 1.20 | 1.23 | 1.26 | 1.30 | 1.33 | 1.39 | 1.45 | 1.50 | 1.56 | 1.61 | 1.66 | 1.71 | | | | | |
| 145 | 0.69 | 0.75 | 0.80 | 0.85 | 0.90 | 0.94 | 0.99 | 1.03 | 1.07 | 1.11 | 1.14 | 1.18 | 1.22 | 1.25 | 1.28 | 1.32 | 1.35 | 1.41 | 1.47 | 1.53 | 1.58 | 1.64 | 1.69 | 1.74 | | | | | |

| Height (cm) | Weight (kg) | | | | | | | | | | | | | | | | | | | | | | | | | | | | |
|---|---|---|---|---|---|---|---|---|---|---|---|---|---|---|---|---|---|---|---|---|---|---|---|---|---|---|---|---|---|
| | 30 | 34 | 38 | 42 | 46 | 50 | 54 | 58 | 62 | 66 | 70 | 74 | 78 | 82 | 86 | 90 | 94 | 98 | 102 | 106 | 110 | 114 | 118 | 122 | | | | | |
| 150 | 1.12 | 1.20 | 1.27 | 1.34 | 1.40 | 1.46 | 1.52 | 1.58 | 1.63 | 1.69 | 1.74 | 1.79 | 1.84 | 1.88 | 1.93 | 1.98 | 2.02 | 2.07 | 2.11 | 2.15 | 2.19 | 2.23 | 2.27 | 2.31 | | | | | |
| 155 | 1.14 | 1.21 | 1.29 | 1.35 | 1.42 | 1.48 | 1.54 | 1.60 | 1.65 | 1.71 | 1.76 | 1.81 | 1.86 | 1.91 | 1.96 | 2.00 | 2.05 | 2.09 | 2.14 | 2.18 | 2.22 | 2.26 | 2.30 | 2.34 | | | | | |
| 160 | 1.15 | 1.23 | 1.30 | 1.37 | 1.44 | 1.50 | 1.56 | 1.62 | 1.68 | 1.73 | 1.78 | 1.84 | 1.89 | 1.94 | 1.98 | 2.03 | 2.08 | 2.12 | 2.17 | 2.21 | 2.25 | 2.29 | 2.34 | 2.38 | | | | | |
| 165 | 1.17 | 1.25 | 1.32 | 1.39 | 1.46 | 1.52 | 1.58 | 1.64 | 1.70 | 1.75 | 1.81 | 1.86 | 1.91 | 1.96 | 2.01 | 2.06 | 2.10 | 2.15 | 2.19 | 2.24 | 2.28 | 2.32 | 2.37 | 2.41 | | | | | |
| 170 | 1.18 | 1.26 | 1.34 | 1.41 | 1.48 | 1.54 | 1.60 | 1.66 | 1.72 | 1.78 | 1.83 | 1.88 | 1.94 | 1.99 | 2.04 | 2.08 | 2.13 | 2.18 | 2.22 | 2.27 | 2.31 | 2.35 | 2.40 | 2.44 | | | | | |
| 175 | 1.20 | 1.28 | 1.35 | 1.43 | 1.49 | 1.56 | 1.62 | 1.68 | 1.74 | 1.80 | 1.85 | 1.91 | 1.96 | 2.01 | 2.06 | 2.11 | 2.16 | 2.20 | 2.25 | 2.30 | 2.34 | 2.38 | 2.43 | 2.47 | | | | | |
| 180 | 1.21 | 1.29 | 1.37 | 1.44 | 1.51 | 1.58 | 1.64 | 1.70 | 1.76 | 1.82 | 1.88 | 1.93 | 1.98 | 2.04 | 2.09 | 2.13 | 2.18 | 2.23 | 2.28 | 2.32 | 2.37 | 2.41 | 2.45 | 2.50 | | | | | |

| Height (cm) | Weight (kg) | | | | | | | | | | | | | | | | | | | | | | | | | | | | |
|---|---|---|---|---|---|---|---|---|---|---|---|---|---|---|---|---|---|---|---|---|---|---|---|---|---|---|---|---|---|
| | 40 | 44 | 48 | 52 | 56 | 60 | 64 | 68 | 72 | 76 | 80 | 84 | 88 | 92 | 96 | 100 | 104 | 108 | 112 | 116 | 120 | 124 | 128 | 132 | | | | | |
| 185 | 1.42 | 1.49 | 1.56 | 1.63 | 1.69 | 1.75 | 1.81 | 1.87 | 1.93 | 1.98 | 2.03 | 2.08 | 2.13 | 2.18 | 2.23 | 2.28 | 2.33 | 2.37 | 2.42 | 2.46 | 2.50 | 2.55 | 2.59 | 2.63 | | | | | |
| 190 | 1.44 | 1.51 | 1.58 | 1.65 | 1.71 | 1.77 | 1.83 | 1.89 | 1.95 | 2.00 | 2.06 | 2.11 | 2.16 | 2.21 | 2.26 | 2.31 | 2.35 | 2.40 | 2.44 | 2.49 | 2.53 | 2.58 | 2.62 | 2.66 | | | | | |
| 195 | 1.45 | 1.53 | 1.60 | 1.67 | 1.73 | 1.79 | 1.85 | 1.91 | 1.97 | 2.02 | 2.08 | 2.13 | 2.18 | 2.23 | 2.28 | 2.33 | 2.38 | 2.43 | 2.47 | 2.52 | 2.56 | 2.60 | 2.65 | 2.69 | | | | | |
| 200 | 1.47 | 1.54 | 1.62 | 1.68 | 1.75 | 1.81 | 1.87 | 1.93 | 1.99 | 2.05 | 2.10 | 2.15 | 2.21 | 2.26 | 2.31 | 2.36 | 2.40 | 2.45 | 2.50 | 2.54 | 2.59 | 2.63 | 2.68 | 2.72 | | | | | |
| 205 | 1.49 | 1.56 | 1.63 | 1.70 | 1.77 | 1.83 | 1.89 | 1.95 | 2.01 | 2.07 | 2.12 | 2.18 | 2.23 | 2.28 | 2.33 | 2.38 | 2.43 | 2.48 | 2.52 | 2.57 | 2.62 | 2.66 | 2.70 | 2.75 | | | | | |
| 210 | 1.50 | 1.58 | 1.65 | 1.72 | 1.79 | 1.85 | 1.91 | 1.97 | 2.03 | 2.09 | 2.14 | 2.20 | 2.25 | 2.30 | 2.36 | 2.41 | 2.45 | 2.50 | 2.55 | 2.60 | 2.64 | 2.69 | 2.73 | 2.77 | | | | | |
| 215 | 1.52 | 1.59 | 1.67 | 1.74 | 1.80 | 1.87 | 1.93 | 1.99 | 2.05 | 2.11 | 2.17 | 2.22 | 2.27 | 2.33 | 2.38 | 2.43 | 2.48 | 2.53 | 2.58 | 2.62 | 2.67 | 2.71 | 2.76 | 2.80 | | | | | |
| 220 | 1.53 | 1.61 | 1.68 | 1.75 | 1.82 | 1.89 | 1.95 | 2.01 | 2.07 | 2.13 | 2.19 | 2.24 | 2.30 | 2.35 | 2.40 | 2.45 | 2.50 | 2.55 | 2.60 | 2.65 | 2.69 | 2.74 | 2.79 | 2.83 | | | | | |

# References


1. Alth G et al. (1973) Aspects of the immunologic treatment of lung cancer. Cancer Chemother Rep 4: 271–274
2. Bomford R (1975) Active specific immunotherapy of mouse methylcholanthrene induced tumors with Corynebacterium parvum and irradiated tumor. Br J Cancer 32: 551–557
3. Fisher B, Rubin H, Sartiano G, Ennis L, Wolmark N (1976) Observations following Corynebacterium parvum administration to patients with advanced malignancy. Cancer 38: 119–130
4. Han T, Takita H (1972) Immunological impairment in bronchogenic carcinoma: a study of lymphocyte response to PHA. Cancer 30: 616–620
5. Humphrey LJ et al. (1971) Immunotherapy for the patients with cancer. Ann Surg 173: 47–54
6. Israel L (1973) Preliminary results of nonspecific immmunotherapy for lung cancer. Cancer Chemother Rep 4: 283–286
7. Kaufmann M, Wirth K, Scheurer J, Zimmermann A, Luscieti P, Stjernsward J (1977) Immunomorphological lymph node changes in patients with operable bronchogenic squamous cell carcinoma. Cancer 39: 2371–2377
8. Khadzhiev S, Kavaklieva-Kimitrova Y (1971) A Treatment of bronchial cancer patients with a water-saline extract of BCG. Vopr Onkol 17: 51–57
9. Krant MJ, Manskopf G, Brandrup CS, Madoff MA (1968) Immunologic alterations in bronchogenic cancer. Sequential study. Cancer 21: 623–631
10. Likhite VV (1976) Experimental cancer immunotherapy: comparison of tumor rejection in F344 rats given live Mycobacterium bovis (strain BCG) and killed Corynebacterium parvum. J Natl Cancer Inst 56: 985–990
11. Ludwig Lung Cancer Cooperative Group (1978) Search for the possible role of "immunotherapy" in operable bronchial non-small cell carcinoma (stage I and II). A phase I study with Corynebacterium parvum intrapleurally. Cancer Immunol Immunother 4: 69–75
12. Matthews MJ (1973) Morphologic classification of bronchogenic carcinoma. Cancer Chemother Rep 4: 299–301
13. McKneally MF, Maver C, Kausel HW (1976) Regional immunotherapy of lung cancer with intrapleural B.C.G. Lancet 1: 377–379
14. Nauts HC, Fowler GA, Bogatko FH (1953) A review of the influence of bacterial infections and of bacterial products (Coley's toxins) on malignant tumors in man. Acta Med Scand 276: 1–103
15. Pimm MV, Baldwin RW (1975) BCG therapy of pleural and peritoneal growth of transplanted rat tumors. Int J Cancer 15: 260–269
16. Pines A (1976) A 5 year controlled study of B.C.G. and radiotherapy for inoperable lung cancer. Lancet 1: 380–381
17. Rees JC, Rossio JL, Wilson HE, Minton JP, Dodd MC (1975) Cellular immunity in neoplasia – antigen and mitagen responses in patients with bronchiogenic carcinoma. Cancer 36: 2010–2015
18. Ruckdeschel JC et al. (1972) Post-operative empyema improves survival in lung cancer. Documentation and analysis of a natural experiment. N Engl J Med 287: 1013–1017
19. Scott MT (1974) Corynebacterium parvum as a therapeutic antitumor agent in mice. II. Local injections. J Natl Cancer Inst 53: 861–865
20. Scott MT (1975) Potentiation of the tumor-specific immune response by Corynebacterium parvum. J Natl Cancer Inst 55: 65–72
21. Scott MT, Bomford R (1976) Comparison of the potentiation of specific tumor immunity in mice by Corynebacterium parvum or BCG. J Natl Cancer Inst 57: 555–559
22. Takita H, Brugarolas A (1973) Adjuvant immunotherapy for bronchogenic carcinoma: preliminary results. Cancer Chemother Rep 4: 293–298
23. Villasor R (1965) The role of immunoblasts in host resistance and immunotherapy of primary sarcoma. Philip Med Assoc 4: 619–632

# Appendix 2. Forms

CONFIRMATION OF REGISTRATION FORM (FORM A)

Institution ___________________________

Person calling ___________________________

☐☐☐☐☐☐☐☐☐☐☐☐☐☐☐☐☐☐☐ Patient's Name (optional)

☐☐☐☐☐☐ Clinical sequence number



___________ Is the patient over 70 years of age? (No only)

___________ Has the patient had any previous malignancy? (No only)

___________ Has the patient been previously treated by irradiation, cytotoxic drugs or immunosuppressants? (No only)

___________ Are there any contraindications to C. Parvum? (No only)

_____/_____/_____ Date of Surgery (d.m.y)

☐☐ ☐☐ ☐☐ Date of Randomization

day   month   year   (must be within 10 days following surgery)

☐ Type of Primary Resection
1- Lobectomy
2- Pneumonectomy or Other ___________
specify

☐ Therapy Assigned
A- Surgery Alone
B- Surgery plus C. Parvum

☐☐☐☐☐ Patient's study number

Follow-Up Forms are Due:

___________________________

___________________________

___________________________

___________________________

___________________________

___________________________

___________________________

___________________________

___________________________

___________________________

Registrar's name

STATISTICAL CENTER
USE ONLY

11/77

CLINICAL and PRE-OPERATIVE FORM (FORM B)          Page 1 of 1

INSTRUCTIONS: Please complete this form after preoperative examinations together with the first column of form F.
Please answer ALL questions on this form. Unless "9-unknown" is provided use "-1" to indicate that an answer is "unknown", "unobtainable", or "not done".

Patient's name ________________________________     Clinic's name ______________________________

L _ _ _ _ _ _ _ _ _ 1 0 0 B 1     Clinic sequence number ____________     Randomization number ____________

INITIAL DATA

1. [____] Year of birth

2. [__] Sex (1-male, 2-female)

3. [___] Current weight (kg)

4. [__] Surface area (M$^2$)

5. [__][__][__] Date of first positive x-ray
   day  month  year

6. [__] Weight loss in previous 6 months (kg)

7. [__] Is there a history of a previous malignancy?
   (1-no, 2-yes, 9-unknown)
   if yes, specify ____________

8. [__] Phrenic paralysis or other nerve dysfunction?
   (1-no, 2-yes, 9-unknown)

9. [__] Associated chronic diseases present?
   (1-no, 2-yes, 9-unknown)
   if yes, specify ____________

Summary of Prior Therapy for Cancer
   (1-no, 2-yes, 9-unknown)

10. [__] Chemotherapy (if yes, describe below)
   ____________________________________

11. [__] Steroids (if yes, describe below)
   ____________________________________

12. [__] Radiation therapy (if yes, describe below)
   ____________________________________

13. [__] Surgery (if yes, describe below)
   ____________________________________

Investigations performed for this trial
   1-not performed
   2-negative, no evidence of cancer or dysfunction
   3-positive, indicative of cancer
   4-positive, indicative of other dysfunction
   5-positive, indicative of cancer and dysfunction
   6-test inconclusive
   9-unknown

14. [__] Laparoscopy
15. [__] Liver scintiscan
16. [__] (mini) laparotomy
17. [__] Ultrasound
18. [__] Pulmonary function tests
19. [__] Mediastinoscopy
20. [__] Bone marrow biopsy

Clinical Signs of Distant Metastases
   1-not involved
   2-positive involvement
   3-questionable involvement
   9-unknown

21. [__] Liver
22. [__] Bone
23. [__] Brain
24. [__] CNS
25. [__] Contralateral lung
26. [__] Extrathoracic lymph node
27. [__] Cervical nodes
28. [__] Supraclavicular nodes
29. [__] Other nodes, specify ____________
30. [__] Other distant metastases, specify ____________

Clinical Evaluation of Disease Stage (before thoracotomy)
   (see reverse side for definitions)

31. [__] T (tumor)
32. [__] N (nodes)
33. [__] M (metastases)

34. [__] Disease stage

Draw site of tumor and all positive nodes as seen from clinical or radiological procedures

Comments:

________________________________________
INVESTIGATOR'S NAME (please print)      DATE

[_________________] STATISTICAL CENTER     INVESTIGATOR: Keep bottom copy and send
                    USE ONLY                            remaining copies to Operations Office     11/77

CLINICAL STAGING (QUESTIONS 31-34)

<u>T - Primary Tumour</u>

0   No evidence of primary tumour.

X   Tumour proven by the presence of malignant cells in bronchopulmonary secretions but not visualised by radiography or bronchoscopy.

1   Tumour 3 cm or less in its greatest dimension, surrounded by lung or visceral pleura and with no evidence of invasion proximal to a lobar bronchus on bronchoscopy.

2   Tumour more than 3 cm in its greatest dimension <u>or</u>

Tumour of any size which, with its associated atalectasis or obstructive pneumonitis, extends to the hilar regions. At bronchoscopy the proximal extent of demonstrable tumour must be at least 2 cm distal to the carina. Any associated atalectasis or obstructive pneumonitis must involve less than an entire lung and there must be no pleural effusion.

3   Tumour of any size with direct extension to adjacent structures such as the chest wall, diaphragm or mediastinum and its contents <u>or</u>

Tumour at bronchoscopy less than 2 cm distal to the carina <u>or</u>

Tumour associated with atalectasis or obstructive pneumonitis of an entire lung or pleural effusion.

<u>N - Regional Lymph Nodes</u>

0   No demonstrable regional lymph nodes.

1   Demonstrable lymph nodes in the homolateral hilar region (including direct extension of primary tumour).

2   Demonstrable lymph nodes in the mediastinum.

<u>M - Distant Metastases</u>

0   No evidence of distant metastases.

1   Distant metastases present including scalene, cervical or contralateral hilar nodes and metastases to brain, bone.

<u>Stage Grouping</u>

| Stage 0 | TX | N0 | M0 |
|---|---|---|---|
| Stage 1 | T0 or TX | N1 | |
| | T1 | N0 or N1 | M0 |
| | T2 | N0 | |
| Stage 2 | T2 | N1 | M0 |
| Stage 3 | Any T3 | Any N2 | Any M1 |

SURGERY FORM (FORM C)                    Page 1 of 1

INSTRUCTIONS: This form is to be filled out after resection.

Please answer ALL questions on this form. Unless "9-unknown" is provided use "-1" to indicate that an answer is "unknown", "unobtainable", or "not done".

Patient's name _______________________________  Clinic's name _____________________________

[ L | | | | | | | | 1 | O | | C | 1 ]   Clinic sequence number _____________  Randomization number _____________

## DETAILS OF SURGERY

1. [ ][ ] [ ][ ] [ ][ ] Date of resection
   day    month   year

2. [ ][ ] Type of primary resection
   10-standard pneumonectomy (right side)
   11-standard pneumonectomy (left side)
   12-standard lobectomy (right upper lobe)
   13-standard lobectomy (right middle lobe)
   14-standard lobectomy (right lower lobe)
   15-standard lobectomy (left upper lobe)
   16-standard lobectomy (left lower lobe)
   17-bilobectomy
   18-wedge or segmental resection
   19-sleeve resection
   20-other, specify _______________________________
   _______________________________
   9-unknown

3. [ ] Extent of primary resection (macroscopically)
   1-radical resection
   2-non-radical resection
   9-unknown

Involvement by Site at Surgery
(1-no, 2-yes, 9-unknown)

4. [ ] Chest wall (ipsilateral)

5. [ ] Diaphragm (ipsilateral)

6. [ ] Mediastinum

7. [ ] Ipsilateral intrapulmonary nodes

8. [ ] Ipsilateral lobar hilar nodes

9. [ ] Ipsilateral lung hilar nodes

10. [ ] Ipsilateral paraesophagel nodes

11. [ ] Ipsilateral subaortic nodes   (left side thoracotomy)

12. [ ] Mediastinal nodes

13. [ ] Other nodes, specify _______________________________

14. [ ] Pleural effusion
    1-present
    2-absent
    9-unknown

## DESCRIPTION OF PRIMARY TUMOR

15. [ ][ ] Location of primary tumor
    10-right upper lobe            16-left upper lobe
    11-right middle lobe           17-left lower lobe
    12-right lower lobe            18-both left lobes
    13-multiple right lobes        19-main bronchus left side
    14-main bronchus right side    20-other,specify _____________
    15-intermediate bronchus        9-unknown

16. [ ][ ] cm x [ ][ ] cm Largest perpendicular diameters
         of primary tumor

17. [ ] Necrosis and/or abscess in primary tumor
    (1-absent, 2-moderate, 3-severe, 9-unknown)

Comments:

---

[ | | | | | | | | ]  STATISTICAL CENTER
                     USE ONLY

INVESTIGATOR'S NAME (please print)    DATE

INVESTIGATOR: Keep bottom copy and send
              remaining copies to Operations Office        11/77

HISTOLOGY and STUDY TREATMENT FORM (FORM D)          Page 1 of 1

INSTRUCTIONS: This form is to be completed after pathological examination of surgical specimens and administration of C. Parvum or Placebo.

Please answer ALL questions on this form. Unless "9-unknown" is provided use "-1" to indicate that an answer is "unknown", "unobtainable", or "not done".

Patient's name ___________________________________        Clinic's name ___________________________________

| L |   |   |   |   | 1 | 0 | 0 | D | 1 |   Clinic sequence number ___________     Randomization number ___________

Histologically examined operational specimens
1-tumor tissue not present
2-tumor tissue present
3-not investigated
9-unknown

1. ☐ Lung with primary tumor

2. ☐ Bronchial resection line

3. ☐ Chest wall

4. ☐ Diaphragm

Nodes

5. ☐ Intersegmental (intrapulmonary)

6. ☐ Lobar hilar

7. ☐ Lung hilar

8. ☐ Para-esophageal

9. ☐ Subaortic (left side thoracotomy)

10. ☐ Mediastinal

11. ☐ Other nodes, specify ___________

12. ☐ Other tissue-specimens, specify ___________

13. ☐ Extra capsular tumor growth of lymph nodes
1-no
2-yes
9-unknown

14. ☐ Cytology of pleural effusion
1-negative
2-positive
9-unknown

Post Histological Evaluation
of Disease Stage
(see reverse side for definitions)

15. ☐ T (tumor)

16. ☐ N (nodes)

17. ☐ M (metastases)

18. ☐ Disease stage

19. ☐☐ Histologic classification

(W.H.O. classification)

10 - squamous cell carcinoma-no further specification
11 - squamous cell carcinoma-highly differentiated
12 - squamous cell carcinoma-moderately differentiated
13 - squamous cell carcinoma-slightly differentiated
20 - small cell carcinoma-no further specification
21 - small cell carcinoma-oval cell structure (oat cell)
22 - small cell carcinoma-transitional or intermediate type
30 - adenocarcinoma-no further specification
31 - adenocarcinoma-well differentiated
32 - adenocarcinoma-moderately well differentiated
33 - adenocarcinoma-poorly differentiated (to include those
     with intracellular mucin without glands)
40 - undifferentiated carcinoma-no further specification
41 - undifferentiated carcinoma-large cell
42 - undifferentiated carcinoma-giant cell
50 - combined squamous and adenocarcinoma or combined
     squamous and small cell carcinoma
60 - other, specify ___________
 9 - unknown

DETAILS OF IMMUNOTHERAPY or Placebo

20. ☐ Randomized therapy
1-surgery alone
2-surgery plus immunotherapy

21. ☐☐ ☐☐ ☐☐ Date of administration of
day  month  year   C. Parvum or Placebo

22. ☐.☐ Administered dose (mg) (if C. Parvum given)

23. ☐ Were thoracic draining tube(s) inserted
at surgery ? (1-no, 2-yes, 9-unknown)

if YES: ☐☐ Number of days in place

24. ☐ Was catheter inserted at
surgery ? (1-no, 2-yes, 9-unknown)

if YES: ☐☐ Number of days in place

25. ☐ Modifications to protocol specifications
for administration
1-no modifications
2-time of administration delayed
3-more than one dose given
4-treatment not administered, specify ___________
5-other, specify ___________
___________
9-unknown

___________________________________
INVESTIGATOR'S NAME (please print)   DATE

| | | | | | | | | | |   STATISTICAL CENTER          INVESTIGATOR: Keep bottom copy and send
                        USE ONLY                                  remaining copies to Operations Office      11/77

POST HISTOLOGICAL STAGING (QUESTIONS 15-18)

## T - Primary Tumour

0   No evidence of primary tumour.

1   Tumor 3 cm or less in its greatest dimension, surrounded by lung or visceral pleura and with no evidence of invasion proximal to a lobar bronchus.

2   Tumor more than 3 cm in its greatest dimension
<u>or</u>

Tumour of any size which, with its associated atalectasis or obstructive pneumonitis, extends to the hilar region.  The proximal extent of tumour must be at least 2 cm distal to the carina. Any associated atalectasis or obstructive pneumonitis must involve less than an entire lung and there must be no pleural effusion.

3   Tumour of any size with direct extension to adjacent structures such as the chest wall, diaphragm or mediastinum and its contents
<u>or</u>

Tumour less than 2 cm distal to the carina
<u>or</u>

Tumour associated with atalectasis or obstructive pneumonitis of an entire lung or pleural effusion.

## N - Regional Lymph Nodes

0   No tumour involvement in lymph nodes.

1   Tumour involvement in lymph nodes in the homolateral hilar region (including direct extension of primary tumour).

2   Tumour involvement in lymph nodes in the mediastinum.

## M - Distant Metastases

0   No evidence of distant metastases.

1   Distant metastases present including scalene, cervical or contralateral hilar nodes and metastases to brain, bone.

## Stage Grouping

| Stage 1 | T0 | N1 | |
|---|---|---|---|
| | T1 | N0 or N1 | M0 |
| | T2 | N0 | |
| Stage 2 | T2 | N1 | M0 |
| Stage 3 | Any T3 | Any N2 | Any M1 |

FOLLOW-UP FORM (FORM E)                                    Page 1 of 1

INSTRUCTIONS: Please complete this form every 3 months together with the fourth column of form F. After 3 years the follow-up
              interval is to be 6 months. Unless "9-unknown" is provided, use "-1" to indicate that an answer is "unknown",
              "unobtainable", or "not done".

Patient's name _________________________________________  Clinic's name _______________________________________

                                                   Clinic sequence number _____________  Randomization number _____________

Follow-up time period

1. from: [  ] [  ] [  ]      (All information entered below is to reflect what has
          day  month  year    occurred during this time period only)

2. to: [  ] [  ] [  ]

3. [  ] Current status of disease
        1-no evidence of disease
        2-positive evidence of disease
        3-possible evidence of disease
        9-unknown

List any events, occuring since last report,
which pertain to course of disease:

EVENT*          Date (d.m.y)                    SITE

4. [  ]    [  ] [  ] [  ]      _______________________________________________

5. [  ]    [  ] [  ] [  ]      _______________________________________________

6. [  ]    [  ] [  ] [  ]      _______________________________________________

7. [  ]    [  ] [  ] [  ]      _______________________________________________

*EVENTS (specify site)
 1-local recurrence (at the site of bronchial stump)
 2-regional recurrence (mediastinal ipsilateral and/or contralateral lymphatic chains)
 3-new regional involvement
 4-distant recurrence
 5-new distant metastases (including contralateral lung and extrathoracic lymph nodes)
 5-other, specify _______________________

Additional therapy during this report period
      (1-no, 2-yes, 9-unknown)              if yes, give details

8. [  ] Surgery ___________________________________________________________________

9. [  ] Radiation therapy _________________________________________________________

10. [  ] Chemotherapy _____________________________________________________________

11. [  ] Other (specify) __________________________________________________________

Complete the following only if the patient
has died or has been lost to follow-up:

12. [  ] Patient status
         2-dead
         3-lost to follow-up, specify reason _______________________

13. [  ] [  ] [  ]   Date of death or date lost to follow-up (d.m.y)      COMMENTS:

Contributing factors of death (1-no, 2-yes, 9-unknown or not applicable)

14. [  ] Local recurrence

15. [  ] Regional recurrence

16. [  ] Distant metastases

17. [  ] Therapy (specify) _______________________

18. [  ] Other (specify) _______________________

19. [  ] Was an autopsy performed?
         (1-no, 2-yes, 9-unknown or not applicable)

                                                      INVESTIGATOR'S NAME (please print)      DATE

[          ] STATISTICAL CENTER        INVESTIGATOR: Keep bottom copy and send
             USE ONLY                                remaining copies to Operations Office      11/77

FLOW SHEET (FORM F)

Page 1 of 1

INSTRUCTIONS: Please submit this form after having completed the appropriate column. Unless "9-unknown" is provided use "-1" to indicate that an answer is "unknown", "unobtainable", or "not done".

Patient's name _______________________________________ Clinic's name ________________________________________

Clinic sequence number _______________ Randomization number _______________

1. ☐☐ ☐☐ ☐☐ Date of visit (d.m.y)

| | Prior to surgical procedures (within one week of surgery) | Before C. Parvum or Placebo (within 24 hours) | After C. Parvum or Placebo (between 24 and 48 hours) | Follow-up visits |
|---|---|---|---|---|
| **BLOOD DIFFERENTIAL  (% of 200 counts)** | | | | |
| 2. Neutrophils (segmented) | ☐☐ | ☐☐ | ☐☐ | ☐☐ |
| 3. Neutrophils (unsegmented) | ☐☐ | ☐☐ | ☐☐ | ☐☐ |
| 4. Eosinophils | ☐☐ | ☐☐ | ☐☐ | ☐☐ |
| 5. Basophils | ☐☐ | ☐☐ | ☐☐ | ☐☐ |
| 6. Lymphocytes | ☐☐ | ☐☐ | ☐☐ | ☐☐ |
| 7. Monocytes | ☐☐ | ☐☐ | ☐☐ | ☐☐ |
| **OTHER HEMATOLOGIC STUDIES** | | | | |
| 8. WBC | ☐☐☐☐☐ | ☐☐☐☐☐ | ☐☐☐☐☐ | ☐☐☐☐☐ |
| 9. PLATELETS | ☐☐☐☐☐☐ | ☐☐☐☐☐☐ | ☐☐☐☐☐☐ | ☐☐☐☐☐☐ |
| 10. ESR (mm in first hour) | ☐☐ | ☐☐ | ☐☐ | ☐☐☐ |
| **LIVER ENZYMES  (1-normal, 2-abnormal,greater than normal, 3-abnormal,less than normal, 9-unknown)** | | | | |
| 11. SGOT | ☐ | | | ☐ |
| 12. SGPT | ☐ | | | ☐ |
| 13. Alkaline phosphatase | ☐ | | | ☐ |
| 14. LAP | ☐ | | | ☐ |
| 15. $\gamma$-GT | ☐ | | | ☐ |
| **COMPLICATIONS AND REACTIONS  (0-none, 1-mild, 2-moderate,  3-severe, 4-life-threatening, 5-lethal, 9-unknown)** | | | | |
| 16. Fever  (>38°c) | ☐ | ☐ | ☐ | ☐ |
| 17. Nausea | ☐ | ☐ | ☐ | ☐ |
| 18. Headache | ☐ | ☐ | ☐ | ☐ |
| 19. Blood pressure change: specify below in comment section | ☐ | ☐ | ☐ | ☐ |
| 20. Infection | ☐ | ☐ | ☐ | ☐ |
| 21. Other, ___________ | ☐ | ☐ | ☐ | ☐ |
| 22. Other, ___________ | ☐ | ☐ | ☐ | ☐ |
| 23. Performance Status (see reverse side for codes) | ☐☐☐ | | | ☐☐☐ |
| **DISEASE INVOLVEMENT  (1-no evidence of disease, 2-positive evidence of disease, 3-questionable evidence of disease, 9-unknown)** | | | | |
| 24. Clinical investigation | ☐ | | | ☐ |
| 25. Lung x-ray (P.A.film) | ☐ | | | ☐ |

COMMENTS:

_______________________________________________
INVESTIGATOR'S NAME (please print)     DATE

STATISTICAL CENTER USE ONLY  ☐☐☐☐☐☐☐☐

INVESTIGATOR: Keep bottom copy and send remaining copies to Operations Office

11/77

Toxicity Criteria

|          | 0        | 1                    | 2                              | 3                          | 4                     |
|----------|----------|----------------------|--------------------------------|----------------------------|-----------------------|
| Fever    | ≤37.5°C  | ≤38° C               | >38° C                         | Severe with Chills (>40° C) | Fever with Hypotension |
| Nausea   | None     | Nausea               | Nausea & Vomiting Controllable | Vomiting Intractable       |                       |
| Headache |          |                      | Moderate Headache              | Severe Headache            |                       |
| Infection | None    | No Active Treatment  | Requires Active Treatment      | Debilitating               | Life Threatening      |

PERFORMANCE STATUS

| 100 | Normal; no complaints, no evidence of disease. |
| 90  | Able to carry on normal activity; minor signs or symptoms of disease. |
| 80  | Normal activity with effort; some signs or symptoms of disease. |
| 70  | Cares for self, unable to carry on normal activity or to do active work. |
| 60  | Requires occasional assistance but is able to care for most of his needs. |
| 50  | Requires considerable assistance and frequent medical care. |
| 40  | Disabled; requires special care and assistance. |
| 30  | Severely disabled; hospitalization is indicated although death not imminent. |
| 20  | Very sick; hospitalization necessary, active supportive treatment is necessary. |
| 10  | Moribund, fatal processes progressing rapidly. |
| 0   | Patient expired. |
| 9   | Unknown. |

Form No. 080          MACROSCOPICAL AND HISTOLOGICAL FORM (FORM P)          Page 1 of 3

INSTRUCTIONS: This form is to be completed and submitted by the participating pathologist at the completion of resection. This form
plus the pathological material for central pathology review should be forwarded to the Operations Office.
Please answer ALL questions on this form. Unless "9-unknown" is provided use "-1" to indicate that an answer is
"unknown", "unobtainable", or "not done".

Patient's name ________________________________     Clinic's name ________________________________

Clinic sequence number ______________     Randomization number ______________

Copies of the local pathology reports should be attached. The following material is being submitted for
central pathology review.

|                                  | Source of Material | Identifying Numbers |
|----------------------------------|--------------------|---------------------|

1. [  ] Number of slides sent
        (enter sources and identifying numbers)

2. [  ] Number of blocks/specimens sent
        (enter sources and identifying numbers)

Name and address of
participating pathologist     ________________________________________________

Histologically examined operational specimens
    1-tumor tissue not present
    2-tumor tissue present
    3-not investigated
    9-unknown

3. [  ] Lung with primary tumor

4. [  ] Bronchial resection line

5. [  ] Chest wall

6. [  ] Diaphragm

Nodes:

7. [  ] Intersegmental (intrapulmonary)

8. [  ] Lobar hilar

9. [  ] Lung hilar

10. [  ] Para-esophageal

11. [  ] Subaortic (left side thoracotomy)

12. [  ] Mediastinal

13. [  ] Other nodes, specify ________________

14. [  ] Other tissue-specimens, specify ________

15. [  ] Extra-capsular tumor growth of lymph nodes
        1-no
        2-yes
        9-unknown

16. [  ] Cytology of pleural effusion
        1-negative
        2-positive
        9-unknown

INVESTIGATOR: Keep last copy and send remaining top copies to Operations Office.                    12/78

Form No.080              MACROSCOPICAL AND HISTOLOGICAL FORM (FORM P)          Page 2 of 3
Patient Name ________________________________          Randomization No. _______________

LOCAL MACROSCOPICAL AND HISTOLOGICAL FINDINGS

Primary Tumor

17.☐☐ Location                                          20.☐ Border
       10-right upper lobe                                     1-circumscribed
       11-right middle lobe                                    2-polycyclic
       12-right lower lobe                                     3-irregular or dissociated
       13-multiple right lobes                                 9-unknown
       14-main bronchus right side
       15-intermediate bronchus                         21.☐ Necrosis
       16-left upper lobe                                      1-absent
       17-left lower lobe                                      2-slight
       18-both left lobes                                      3-moderate
       19-main bronchus left side                              4-severe
       20-other, specify _______________                      9-unknown
        9-unknown
                                                        22.☐ Hemorrhage
18.  Lung Segment Resection   (International                   1-absent
     1-not resected              Classification)              2-slight
     2-completely resected                                     3-moderate
     3-partially resected                                      4-severe
     9-unknown                                                 9-unknown

              Right Upper Lobe                          23.☐ Level of invasion
                                                               1-to inner border of bronchial cartilage
☐  1.Apical                                                    2-to outer border of bronchial cartilage
                                                               3-invasion of alveolar lung tissue
☐  2.Posterior                                                 9-unknown

☐  3.Anterior                                           24.☐ Invasions of vessels
              Middle Lobe                                      1-no invasion
                                                               2-invasion of blood vessels
☐  4.Lateral                                                   3-invasion of lymph vessels
                                                               4-invasion of both blood and lymph vessels
☐  5.Medial                                                    5-lymphangiosis carcinomatosa s. neoplastica
              Right Lower Lobe                                 6-invasion of blood vessels and
                                                                 lymphangiosis carcinomatosa
☐  6.Apical                                                    7-other, specify ___________________
                                                               9-unknown
☐  7.Medial basal
                                                        25.☐ Invasion of pleura visceralis
☐  8.Anterior basal                                            1-no
                                                               2-yes
☐  9.Lateral basal                                             9-unknown

☐  10.Posterior basal                                  26.☐ Differentiation
              Left Upper Lobe                                  1-well differentiated
                                                               2-moderately differentiated
☐  1.Apical                                                    3-poorly differentiated
                                                               4-no exact grading possible
☐  2.Posterior                                                 9-unknown

☐  3.Anterior                                          27.☐☐ Histologic classification

☐  4.Superior                                              (W.H.O. classification)

☐  5.Inferior                                          10 - squamous cell carcinoma-no further specification
              Left Lower Lobe                          11 - squamous cell carcinoma-highly differentiated
                                                       12 - squamous cell carcinoma-moderately differentiated
☐  6.Apical                                            13 - squamous cell carcinoma-slightly differentiated
                                                       20 - small cell carcinoma-no further specification
☐  8.Anterobasal                                       21 - small cell carcinoma-oval cell structure (oat cell)
                                                       22 - small cell carcinoma-transitional or intermediate type
☐  9.Lateral basal                                     30 - adenocarcinoma-no further specification
                                                       31 - adenocarcinoma-well differentiated
☐  10.Posterior basal                                  32 - adenocarcinoma-moderately well differentiated
                                                       33 - adenocarcinoma-poorly differentiated (to include
19. Size:largest perpendicular diameters                    those with intracellular mucin without glands)
    of primary tumor                                   40 - undifferentiated carcinoma-no further specification
                                                       41 - undifferentiated carcinoma-large cell
☐☐.☐ cm X ☐☐.☐ cm (unfixed)                            42 - undifferentiated carcinoma-giant cell
                                                       50 - combined squamous and adenocarcinoma or combined
☐☐.☐ cm X ☐☐.☐ cm (fixed)                                   squamous and small cell carcinoma
                                                       60 - other, specify ___________________________
                                                        9 - unknown

INVESTIGATOR: Keep last copy and send remaining top copies to Operations Office.          12/78

Form No.080          MACROSCOPICAL AND HISTOLOGICAL FORM (FORM P)          Page 3 of 3
Patient Name ________________________          Randomization No. ________________

INVOLVEMENT OF LOCO-REGIONAL LYMPH NODES

| | Lung Periphery (Segmental) | Lobar Hilus | Lung Hilus | Mediastinum (paratracheal, subcarinal [trachea bifuracation] tracheobronchial angle: ipsilateral and/or contralateral) | Subaortic region (left side thoracotomy only) | Paraoesophageal Region | Other intrathoracal specify ________ |
|---|---|---|---|---|---|---|---|
| Number Examined • | ☐☐ | ☐☐ | ☐☐ | ☐☐ | ☐☐ | ☐☐ | ☐☐ |
| Number Involved • | ☐☐ | ☐☐ | ☐☐ | ☐☐ | ☐☐ | ☐☐ | ☐☐ |
| Number with Extracapsular growth • | ☐☐ | ☐☐ | ☐☐ | ☐☐ | ☐☐ | ☐☐ | ☐☐ |

• Enter number - if countable
  Enter 98 - if diffused
  Enter -1 - if unknown

Comments:

INVESTIGATOR'S NAME (please print) _______________ DATE ______

STATISTICAL CENTER USE ONLY          INVESTIGATOR: Keep bottom copy and send
                                      remaining copies to Operations Office          12/78

Form No. 082                 CENTRAL PATHOLOGY REVIEW FORM (FORM R)                Page 1 of 1

INSTRUCTIONS: This form is to be completed and submitted by the Central Pathologist upon completion of the central review. If there is insufficient material for central review, the top part of this form is to function as a request for additional material.
   Please answer ALL questions on this form. Unless "9-unknown" is provided use "-1" to indicate that an answer is "unknown", "unobtainable", or "not done".

Patient's name ___________________________________________   Clinic's name ________________________________

[L | | | | | | | | | 1 | | R | 1 ]   Clinic sequence number _______________   Randomization number _______________

☐ Sufficient material for review received?
   1-no, specify below
   2-yes

____________________________________________________________________________

____________________________________________________________________________

____________________________________________________________________________

If the material is not sufficient, the review should stop at this point and this form returned to the participant as a request for further material.

[☐☐] [☐☐] [☐☐] Date sufficient material received
 day   month  year

CENTRAL REVIEW RESULTS

| Histologic Classification* | Differ- entiation** | Reviewer's Initials | Name of Reviewer |

☐☐   ☐   ☐☐☐ ___________
☐☐   ☐   ☐☐☐ ___________
☐☐   ☐   ☐☐☐ ___________
☐☐   ☐   Final Diagnosis

Comments:

• Histologic classification

   (W.H.O. classification)

   10 – squamous cell carcinoma-no further specification
   11 – squamous cell carcinoma-highly differentiated
   12 – squamous cell carcinoma-moderately differentiated
   13 – squamous cell carcinoma-slightly differentiated
   20 – small cell carcinoma-no further specification
   21 – small cell carcinoma-oval cell
        structure (oat cell)
   22 – small cell carcinoma-transitional or
        intermediate type
   30 – adenocarcinoma-no further specification
   31 – adenocarcinoma-well differentiated
   32 – adenocarcinoma-moderately well differentiated
   33 – adenocarcinoma-poorly differentiated (to include
        those with intracellular mucin without glands)
   40 – undifferentiated carcinoma-no further
        specification
   41 – undifferentiated carcinoma-large cell
   42 – undifferentiated carcinoma-giant cell
   50 – combined squamous and adenocarcinoma or combined
        squamous and small cell carcinoma
   60 – other, specify ________________________________
    9 – unknown

   **Differentiation
   1-well differentiated
   2-moderately differentiated
   3-poorly differentiated
   4-no exact grading possible
   9-unknown

[ | | | | | | | | ] STATISTICAL CENTER USE ONLY

_______________________________________________
                    INVESTIGATOR'S NAME (please print)        DATE

INVESTIGATOR: Keep bottom copy and send
             remaining copies to Operations Office        12/78

Form No. 085                                                                 Page 1 of 1

ELIGIBILITY and THERAPY ADMINISTRATION EVALUATION FORM (FORM V1)

INSTRUCTIONS: This form will be initiated by the Statistical Center when complete initial patient forms are received, and will be forwarded to the study coordinator for review.

Please answer ALL questions on this form. Unless "9-unknown" is provided use "-1" to indicate that an answer is "unknown", "unobtainable", or "not done".

Patient's name ___________________________     Clinic's name ___________________________

L [ ][ ][ ][ ][ ][ ][ ][ ][1][0][0][V][1]   Clinic sequence number __________   Randomization number __________

|  | Statistical Center | Study Coordinator |
|---|---|---|
| 1.Was the patient eligible? (1-no, 2-yes) | ☐ | ☐ |

Eligibility Review

(1-not eligible,2-eligible,3-questionable)

|  | Statistical Center | Study Coordinator |
|---|---|---|
| 2.Study entry date | ☐ | ☐ |
| 3.Histology | ☐ | ☐ |
| 4.Post histologic Stage I or II disease | ☐ | ☐ |
| 5.Acceptable surgical procedure | ☐ | ☐ |
| 6.Age  ( < 70) | ☐ | ☐ |
| 7.Prior malignancy | ☐ | ☐ |
| 8.Prior irradiation, or cytotoxic drugs | ☐ | ☐ |
| 9.Prior immunosuppressants | ☐ | ☐ |
| 10.Medical unsuitability | ☐ | ☐ |
| 11.Positive mediastinoscopy or mediastinal nodes | ☐ | ☐ |
| 12.Neoplastic growth at resection line | ☐ | ☐ |
| 13.Pleural exudate | ☐ | ☐ |
| 14.Other, specify _______________ | ☐ | ☐ |

Therapy Administration

| 15.Modifications to protocol specifications | ☐ | ☐ |
|---|---|---|

1-no modification
2-acceptable modification, specify below
3-unacceptable modification, specify below
9-cannot determine

Comments:

___________________________  _______     ___________________________  _______
STATISTICAL CENTER (please print)  DATE     STUDY COORDINATOR (please print)  DATE

[ ][ ][ ][ ][ ][ ][ ][ ][ ]  STATISTICAL CENTER USE ONLY     INVESTIGATOR: Keep bottom copy and send remaining copies to Operations Office     12/78

Form No. 081                   AUTOPSY FORM (FORM Z)                 Page 1 of 2

INSTRUCTIONS: This form is to be completed and submitted by the pathologist after autopsy. A copy of the local autopsy form should be included.

Please answer ALL questions on this form. Unless "9-unknown" is provided use "-1" to indicate that an answer is "unknown", "unobtainable", or "not done".

Patient's name ________________________________ Clinic's name ______________________________

Clinic sequence number __________ Randomization number __________

1. ☐☐ ☐☐ ☐☐ Date of death
   day  month  year

2. ☐☐ ☐☐ ☐☐ Date of autopsy
   day  month  year

3. ☐ Main cause of death
    1-recurrence (loco/regional) of lung cancer
    2-recurrence (distant metastases) of lung cancer
    3-recurrence (both loco/regional and distant metastases) of lung cancer
    4-probable true second lung cancer (attach further comments)
    5-cardiopulmonary failure
    6-other main cause of death, specify ______________________
    9-unknown

Contributing Factors of Death
(1-no, 2-yes, 9-unknown or not applicable)

4. ☐ Local recurrence

5. ☐ Regional recurrence

6. ☐ Distant metastases

7. ☐ Therapy (specify) __________________________

8. ☐ Other (specify) __________________________

If there was local recurrence, answer question 9.

9. ☐   1-same histological type and degree of differentiation as primary tumor
    2-same histological type but not the same degree of differentiation
    3-other histological type
    9-unknown
    if 2 or 3, specify ____________________________

If there was regional recurrence, answer question 10.

10. ☐   1-same histological type and degree of differentiation as primary tumor
    2-same histological type but not the same degree of differentiation
    3-other histological type
    9-unknown
    if 2 or 3, specify ____________________________

Form No..081       AUTOPSY FORM (FORM 2)       Page 2 of 2

Patient Name ______________________      Randomization No. ______________

If distant metastases were present, answer questions 11 through 22.
1-same histological type and degree of differentiation as primary tumor
2-same histological type but not the same degree of differentiation
3-other histological type
9-unknown
if 2 or 3, specify in the column on the right

Histologic Classification

11. ☐ Ipsilateral lung (site of bronchial stump excluded) ______________

12. ☐ Contralateral lung and/or adjacent lymph nodes ______________

13. ☐ Contralateral chest wall and/or diaphragm ______________

14. ☐ Liver ______________

15. ☐ Bony skeleton, specify: ________________________ ______________

16. ☐ Brain ______________

17. ☐ Adrenal glands ______________

18. ☐ Kidney ______________

19. ☐ Retroperitoneal lymph nodes ______________

20. ☐ Pancreas ______________

21. ☐ Other extrathoracal lymph nodes, specify: __________ ______________

22. ☐ Other distant organs/tissues, specify: __________ ______________

COMMENTS:

INVESTIGATOR'S NAME (please print)    DATE

STATISTICAL CENTER USE ONLY      INVESTIGATOR: Keep bottom copy and send remaining copies to Operations Office      12/78

# *Appendix 3. Example of Data Request*

*Form Titles*

B – Clinical and pre-operative; C – Surgery; D – Histology and study treatment; E – Follow-up; F – Flow sheet

Please submit the following data to the operations office by March 1, 1977
(see cover letter for explanation)

Institution: Bern

| Lung | | | Form (see above for description) | Scheduled date |
|------|------|-----------|------|----------------|
| No. | Name | C.S. no.[a] | | |
| 4 | Green, James | 00045 | E | 7/10/77 |
| | | | E | 7/1/78 |
| | | | F | Pre surgery |
| | | | F | 7/10/77 |
| | | | F | 7/1/78 |
| 11 | White, John | 00053 | E | 21/10/77 |
| | | | E | 21/1/78 |
| | | | F | 21/10/77 |
| | | | F | 21/1/78 |
| 25 | Brown, Mary | 00154 | E | 5/11/77 |
| | | | E | 5/2/78 |
| | | | F | Post-treatment or placebo |
| | | | F | 5/11/77 |
| | | | F | 5/2/78 |
| 40 | Black, Arthur | 00431 | B | Study entry |
| | | | C | Study entry |
| | | | D | Post-treatment or placebo |
| | | | F | Pre-surgery |
| | | | F | Pre-treatment or placebo |
| | | | F | Post-treatment or placebo |

[a] C.S. no., Clinic sequence number

# Appendix 4. Example of Patient Listing

Bern

| Case no. | Name | C.S. no. | Assigned treatment | Date entered | Date of recur- rence | Status | Date of last contact or death | Remarks |
|---|---|---|---|---|---|---|---|---|
| 4 | Green, James | 00045 | Placebo | 7-7-77 | | Alive | 17-7-77 | |
| 11 | White, John | 00053 | *C. parvum* | 21-7-77 | | Alive | 1-8-77 | |
| 18 | Jones, Harold | 00099 | *C. parvum* | 1-8-77 | | Alive | 1-11-77 | |
| 25 | Brown, Mary | 00154 | Placebo | 8-9-77 | | Alive | 15-12-77 | |
| 34 | Marx, William | 00314 | *C. parvum* | 29-9-77 | | Dead | 5-10-77 | No treatment |
| 40 | Black, Arthur | 00431 | Placebo | 20-11-77 | | Alive | 30-11-77 | |
| 53 | Johnson, Joseph | 00619 | *C. parvum* | 2-12-77 | | Alive | 12-12-77 | |
| 61 | Martin, George | 00658 | *C. parvum* | 20-12-77 | | Alive | 20-12-77 | |

# Appendix 5. Participant Forms Submission Log

*Example*

Name: Mary Smith      Clinical sequence no.: 078-22-77      Case no.: 3

Treatment: Surgery and immunotherapy

Date of surgery: 1/9/77

| Parameters | Prior surgery | Before *C. parvum* or placebo (within 24 h) | After *C. parvum* or placebo (between 24–48 h) | Every 3 months |
|---|---|---|---|---|
| History and physical exam | × | | | |
| Clinical examination | × | | | × |
| Lung X-ray (P.A. and lateral) | × | | | × |
| Performance status | × | | | × |
| Blood diff. and hematologic studies (Neutrophils [seg], neutrophils [unseg], eosinophils, basophils, lymphocytes, monocytes, WBC, platelets and erythrocyte sedimentation rate) | × | × | × | × |
| Liver enzymes (SGOT, SGPT, alkaline phosphatase, LAP, and $\gamma$-GT) | ×[a] | | | × |
| Mediastinoscopy | × | | | |
| Bone marrow biopsy | [b] | | | |

[a] If suspect for liver metastases, see protocol for required tests

[b] If > 10 kg weight loss in previous 6 months, bone marrow biopsy is required

| Forms | Date sent | Follow-up forms are due: | Date sent |
|---|---|---|---|
| Clinical and pre-operative form (B) | | | |
| Flow sheet (F) | ———— | ———— | ———— |
| Surgery form (C) | ———— | ———— | ———— |
| Flow sheet (F) within 24 h prior to *C. parvum* or placebo | ———— | ———— | ———— |
| Flow sheet (F) between 24–48 h after *C. parvum* or placebo | ———— | ———— | ———— |
| Study treatment and histology form (D) | ———— | ———— | ———— |

# Appendix 6. Operations Office Patient Log

Patient Log. Please enter date each form was received in the corresponding column

| Study no. | Patient name Clinic sequence no. Institute | Pre-surgery Form F | Form B | Form C | Before C. *par-vum* or placebo Form F | After C. *par-vum* or placebo Form F | Form D | Form E and F (1st, 2nd, 3rd) | Form E and F (4th, 5th, 6th) | Form E and F | Form E and F | Form E and F | Form E and F | Form E and F | Form E and F | Form P | Form Z |
|---|---|---|---|---|---|---|---|---|---|---|---|---|---|---|---|---|---|
|  |  |  |  |  |  |  |  |  |  |  |  |  |  |  |  |  |  |
|  |  |  |  |  |  |  |  |  |  |  |  |  |  |  |  |  |  |
|  |  |  |  |  |  |  |  |  |  |  |  |  |  |  |  |  |  |
|  |  |  |  |  |  |  |  |  |  |  |  |  |  |  |  |  |  |
|  |  |  |  |  |  |  |  |  |  |  |  |  |  |  |  |  |  |
|  |  |  |  |  |  |  |  |  |  |  |  |  |  |  |  |  |  |
|  |  |  |  |  |  |  |  |  |  |  |  |  |  |  |  |  |  |
|  |  |  |  |  |  |  |  |  |  |  |  |  |  |  |  |  |  |
|  |  |  |  |  |  |  |  |  |  |  |  |  |  |  |  |  |  |

# *Appendix 7. Sample Page of Randomization List*

Basel, Pneumonectomy

| Patient name (or number) | Rand. number | Rand. date | Conf. form | Therapy |
|---|---|---|---|---|
| 1. | | | | A |
| 2. | | | | B |
| 3. | | | | A |
| 4. | | | | B |
| 5. | | | | B |
| 6. | | | | A |
| 7. | | | | B |
| 8. | | | | A |
| 9. | | | | B |
| 10. | | | | A |
| 11. | | | | B |
| 12. | | | | A |
| 13. | | | | B |
| 14. | | | | A |
| 15. | | | | B |
| 16. | | | | A |
| 17. | | | | A |
| 18. | | | | A |
| 19. | | | | B |
| 20. | | | | B |
| 21. | | | | A |
| 22. | | | | A |
| 23. | | | | B |
| 24. | | | | B |

Treatment codes: A = surgery plus placebo;  B = surgery plus *C. parvum*

## Appendix 8. Sample Data File

```
L771100001100A1B0121Green  Henry            00001070777
L771100001100B1    192410601518037700111111111111221111111111111001
L771100001100C1    30067715121111111111121602021
L771100001100D1    2111211111111191001102070777072072071
L771100001100V1    2
L771100001101F1    290677-1-1-1-1-1-1004600              -101799199000008810012
L771100001102F1    010777-1-1-1-1-1-1-1      -1          -1 -1      0000088
L771100001103F1    070777-1-1-1-1-1-1-1      -1          -1 -1      1001088
L771100002100A1A0021Brown  John          75812070777
L771100002100B1     1915106218260577-1112111111112211111111111001
L771100002100C1    0107771511111111111111603031
L771100002100D1    2111111111111191001131070777-12042071
L771100002100V1    2
L771100002101E1    1107772509771                                1118
L771100002101F1    200677620401012507006500017000007111910000000010033
L771100002102F1    040777650900011708009100021500000 1      0000000
L771100002103F1    110777610903032004008300021500004 9      0000000
L771100002104F1    250977520000013611004300031400001211111000012808011
L771100003100A1A0062White  James          62177070777
L771100003100B1     19241078200905770011211111111451111111111121001
L771100003100C1    28067711111222128292172-7-2-21
L771100003100D1    21212222111119210241107077-7-11     2091
L771100003100T1    Q eligibility positive para-esophageal nodes
L771100003100V1    1
L771100003101E1    1207772010771
L771100003101F1    090577590304003301006900              -106821199888888809012
L771100003102F11
L771100003103F1    11077764000301240800770 0      -1068      8888888
L771100003104F1    201077640402022105007800025500002311111000000009011
```

Forms received

*Appendix 9. Statistical Center Forms Log*

| Patient Clinic, no. Treatment | Study case (no.) | Date randomized | Institution | B | C | D | 01 F | 02 F | 03 F | FOLLOW-UPS: FORMS E and F<br>Legend: o Month on study<br>x E form received<br># F form seqquence | Death forms E | Z |
|---|---|---|---|---|---|---|---|---|---|---|---|---|
| Smith Harvey 415-77 A | 21 | 8-2-77 | 12 | x | x | x | x | x | x | | | |
| Jones John 0208242 A | 22 | 8-3-77 | 1 | x | x | x | x | x | x | ③ 04 | | |
| Brown Mark 23000 B | 23 | 8-4-77 | 13 | x | x | x | x | x | x | ③ 04 | | |
| Green Abel 18268 A | 24 | 8-4-77 | 7 | x | x | x | x | x | x | ③ 04 | | |
| Black Robert 5 A | 25 | 8-5-77 | 4 | x | x | x | x | x | x | | | |
| White Carl 48477 B | 26 | 8-8-77 | 12 | x | x | x | x | x | x | | | |
| Hart Homer 48577 B | 27 | 8-8-77 | 12 | x | x | x | x | x | x | | | |
| Crown James 23415 B | 28 | 8-8-77 | 13 | x | x | x | x | x | x | ③ 04 | | |
| Dodd Thomas 6 B | 29 | 8-9-77 | 4 | x | x | x | x | x | x | | | |
| Finn Frederick 74502 393 B | 30 | 8-10-77 | 2 | x | x | x | x | x | x | | | |

Totals by month on study:

| | 1 A | 1 B | 2 A | 2 B | 4 A | 4 B | 5 A | 5 B | 6 A | 6 B | 7 A | 7 B | 8 A | 8 B | 9 A | 9 B | 10 A | 10 B | 11 A | 11 B | 12 A | 12 B | 13 A | 13 B | Total A | Total B |
|---|---|---|---|---|---|---|---|---|---|---|---|---|---|---|---|---|---|---|---|---|---|---|---|---|---|---|
| | 1 | | 2 | 1 | 2 | 1 | | | 3 | 2 | 1 | 2 | 1 | | | | | | 1 | 1 | | 1 | 2 | | 13 | 7 |
| | 2 | | 2 | 1 | 3 | 2 | | | 3 | 2 | 2 | 2 | 1 | | | | | | 1 | 1 | 1 | 3 | 2 | 2 | 17 | 13 |

*Appendix 10. Example of an Interim Statistical Analysis*

**Study 1**
Biostatistician's report
February 1979

Project Title

Locoregional and systemic immunostimulation as adjuvant therapy in radical resected bronchogenic squamous cell carcinoma, adenocarcinoma and large cell carcinoma.

Patient Population

Patients with histologically proven squamous cell carcinoma, adenocarcinoma or large cell carcinoma and classified post surgically as $T_1N_0M_0$, $T_2N_0M_0$, $T_1N_1M_0$, or $T_2N_1M_0$.

Schema

(Stratify by type of surgery)

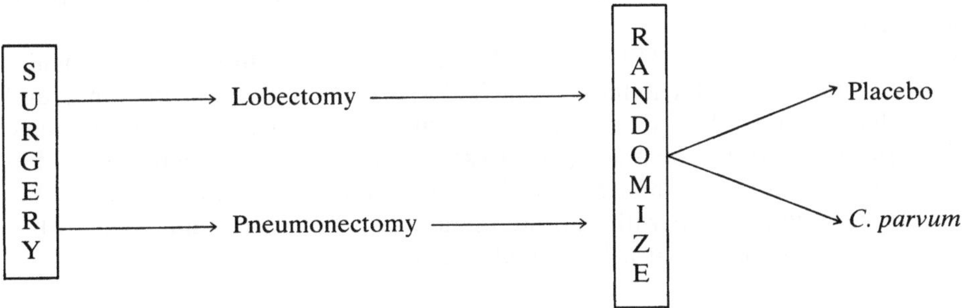


*C. parvum:*

7 mg intrapleurally once between days 6 and 10 postoperatively.

Study Activated

1 July 1977.

Entry Terminated

2 February 1979.

Total Accrual

475 patients.

**Summary and Study Status**

Entry onto Study 1, comparing intrapleural *C. parvum* versus placebo, was terminated 2 February 1979 after 475 patients had been entered. Study 2, comparing intrapleural plus intravenous *C. parvum* versus intrapleural BCG versus placebo, was activated on 5 February 1979.

This is an interim report on the progress of Study 1. Plans are under way for a summer 1979 analysis of the initial patient information, therapy administration, and therapy complications. It is anticipated that approximately 2 years of follow-up will be required before it will be possible to make definitive comparisons of the treatments with regard to disease-free interval or survival. However, it is possible to identify a few high-risk groups. Preliminary indications are that surgical stage, type of resection, and degree of differentiation are prognostic factors. Central histology review is a very promising area and it is recommended that efforts be continued to gather and evaluate this material.

More complications (especially fever and pleuritic or chest pain) have been observed for the patients receiving *C. parvum*. A fever of greater than 38° C was observed in 37% of the patients assigned to *C. parvum* as opposed to 9% of the patients assigned to placebo.


**Administrative Information**

Table 2 presents patient accrual and case status by treatment. An ineligible case is one in which there is sufficient ground for the determination of ineligibility according to protocol criteria.

There were 52 ineligible cases; 34 had Stage III disease, 9 had tumor at the bronchial resection line, 7 had small cell carcinoma, one had a second subpleural carcinoma, and one did not have cancer. Entry onto this study did not require that the histologic diagnosis of surgical material be made prior to study entry. This has been modified in the next study and should dramatically reduce the number of ineligible cases. Six patients were cancelled; three with chronic pneumonia, not carcinoma, two with a nonlung primary, and one with a bronchial adenoma.


**Table 2.** Distribution of patients by case status

|  | Treatment | | |
|---|---|---|---|
|  | Surgery plus placebo | Surgery plus *C. parvum* | Total |
| Patients entered | 236 | 239 | 475 |
|   Cancelled | 3 | 3 | 6 |
|   B, C, and D forms not received | 20 | 10 | 30 |
|   Ineligible patients | 26 | 26 | 52 |
| Properly entered and eligible | 187 | 200 | 387 |
|   No follow-up data available | 36 | 37 | 73 |
| Cases analyzed | 151 | 163 | 314 |

**Table 3.** Patients entered by month by institution

| | 1977 | | | 1978 | | | | | | 1979 | Total |
|---|---|---|---|---|---|---|---|---|---|---|---|
| | July/ Aug | Sept/ Oct | Nov/ Dec | Jan/ Feb | Mar/ Apr | May/ June | Jul/ Aug | Sept/ Oct | Nov/ Dec | Jan/ Feb | |
| Aarhus | 3 | 4 | 8 | 2 | 2 | 2 | 4 | 7 | 3 | 2 | 37 |
| Basel | 4 | 4 | 3 | 3 | 2 | 6 | 2 | 0 | 3 | 0 | 27 |
| Bern (Insel) | 7 | 5 | 3 | 7 | 6 | 7 | 5 | 4 | 1 | 0 | 45 |
| Bern (Tiefenau) | 0 | 2 | 1 | 0 | 2 | 1 | 2 | 0 | 1 | 1 | 10 |
| Essen | 7 | 5 | 5[a] | 3 | 5 | 9 | 7 | 7 | 5 | 4 | 57 |
| Heidelberg | 5 | 4 | 11 | 10 | 13 | 8 | 11 | 5 | 5 | 7 | 79 |
| Ljubljana | 2 | 9 | 7 | 8 | 6 | 4 | 5 | 8 | 8 | 6 | 63 |
| Lowenstein | 1 | 2 | 0 | 1 | 2 | 1 | 4 | 0 | 3 | 1 | 15 |
| Oslo | 0 | 1 | 7 | 6 | 8 | 4 | 5 | 4 | 5 | 2 | 42 |
| Solothurn | 2 | 3 | 2 | 2 | 1 | 0 | 1 | 1 | 0 | 0 | 12 |
| Stockholm | 5 | 1 | 7 | 1 | 9 | 2 | 0 | 2 | 5 | 0 | 32 |
| Vienna | 4 | 2 | 8 | 4 | 10 | 6 | 5 | 11 | 5 | 1 | 56 |
| Total | 40 | 42 | 62 | 47 | 66 | 50 | 51 | 49 | 44 | 24 | 475 |

[a] Entry stopped temporarily due to infection in the clinic

**Table 4.** Case status by institution

| | Patients cancelled | B, C, and D forms not received | Ineligible | No Follow-up data available | Analyzable cases (%) | Total entered |
|---|---|---|---|---|---|---|
| Aarhus | 1 | 1 | 1 | 5 | 29 (78) | 37 |
| Basel | 1 | 0 | 2 | 2 | 22 (81) | 27 |
| Bern (Insel) | 1 | 1 | 7 | 7 | 29 (64) | 45 |
| Bern (Tiefenau) | 0 | 1 | 2 | 1 | 6 (60) | 10 |
| Essen | 0 | 10 | 10 | 5 | 32 (56) | 57 |
| Heidelberg | 2 | 7 | 10 | 19 | 41 (52) | 79 |
| Ljubljana | 1 | 6 | 9 | 6 | 41 (65) | 63 |
| Lowenstein | 0 | 0 | 2 | 4 | 9 (60) | 15 |
| Oslo | 0 | 2 | 5 | 5 | 30 (71) | 42 |
| Solothurn | 0 | 0 | 2 | 1 | 9 (75) | 12 |
| Stockholm | 0 | 1 | 1 | 9 | 21 (66) | 32 |
| Vienna | 0 | 1 | 1 | 9 | 45 (80) | 56 |
| Total | 6 | 30 | 52 | 73 | 314 (66) | 475 |

Accrual in the trial has been approximately 25 patients per months. Table 3 gives case entry by time for each of the participants.

Table 4 presents the case status of the patients entered by each participant. A short delay in the receipt of forms of patients recently randomized should be expected.

The remainder of this report will be based on the 314 analyzable cases.

## Patient and Disease Characteristics

Table 5 presents the distribution of patients by age, sex, stage, participant histology, central histology, and central histologic differentiation versus treatment. The treatments appear to be well balanced with regard to all of these factors except stage. *C. parvum* appears to have a higher percentage of $T_1N_0M_0$ patients than the placebo group. Eventual treatment comparisons must take this imbalance into account. Central histology review results are available for 52% (164 of 314) of the analyzable cases.

**Table 5.** Patient and disease characteristics

| Characteristic | Level | Surgery plus placebo | Surgery plus *C. parvum* | Total no. of patients | Percentage of patients |
|---|---|---|---|---|---|
| Age | < 50 years | 21 | 27 | 48 | 15 |
|  | 50−59 years | 58 | 66 | 124 | 40 |
|  | 60−70 years | 71 | 70 | 141 | 45 |
| Sex | Male | 133 | 140 | 273 | 87 |
|  | Female | 18 | 23 | 41 | 13 |
| Surgical stage | $T_1N_0M_0$ | 47 | 61 | 108 | 34 |
|  | $T_2N_0M_0$ | 62 | 66 | 128 | 41 |
|  | $T_1N_1M_0$ | 11 | 10 | 21 | 7 |
|  | $T_2N_1M_0$ | 31 | 26 | 57 | 18 |
| Participant histology | Squamous cell | 103 | 102 | 205 | 65 |
|  | Adenocarcinoma | 28 | 36 | 64 | 20 |
|  | Large cell | 13 | 20 | 33 | 11 |
|  | Other | 7 | 5 | 12 | 4 |
| Central histology (164 cases, 52%) | Squamous cell | 54 | 48 | 102 | 62 |
|  | Small cell | 0 | 4 | 4 | 2 |
|  | Adenocarcinoma | 15 | 18 | 33 | 20 |
|  | Large cell | 9 | 4 | 13 | 8 |
|  | Other | 5 | 7 | 12 | 7 |
| Central histologic differentiation | Well differentiated | 23 | 23 | 46 | 30 |
|  | Moderately differentiated | 31 | 33 | 64 | 42 |
|  | Poorly differentiated | 23 | 21 | 44 | 29 |

## Treatment Administration and Complications

Table 6 gives information concerning the surgical procedures and administration of *C. parvum* or placebo.

Complications were recorded subjectively as either none, mild, moderate, severe, life threatening, or lethal. In this manner, complications of different types may be summarized and an overall idea of the level of complications for each patient may be obtained. Table 7 presents a comparison of "worst degree of complication" between the treatment regimens. The "worst degree of complication" refers to the most severe degree of complication experienced by each patient.

**Table 6.** Surgical procedures and administration of placebo or *C. parvum*

| | Surgery plus placebo | Surgery plus *C. parvum* | Overall |
|---|---|---|---|
| | *n (%)* | *n (%)* | *n (%)* |
| Type of resection | | | |
| Pneumonectomy | 41 (27) | 41 (25) | 82 (26) |
| Lobectomy | 90 (60) | 98 (60) | 188 (60) |
| Bilobectomy (upper lobe remaining) | 3 (2) | 7 (4) | 10 (3) |
| Bilobectomy (lower lobe remaining) | 6 (4) | 2 (1) | 8 (3) |
| Other[a] | 11 (7) | 15 (9) | 26 (8) |
| Draining tubes | | | |
| Not used | 16 (11) | 18 (11) | 34 (11) |
| Used 1−5 days | 73 (48) | 72 (44) | 145 (46) |
| Used 6−10 days | 50 (33) | 60 (37) | 110 (35) |
| Used 11−15 days | 6 (4) | 9 (6) | 15 (5) |
| Used more than 15 days | 5 (3) | 4 (3) | 9 (3) |
| Used (duration not specified) | 1 (1) | 0 | 1 (<1) |
| Catheter | | | |
| Not used | 3 (2) | 11 (7) | 14 (5) |
| Used 1−5 days | 12 (8) | 2 (1) | 14 (5) |
| Used 6−10 days | 121 (80) | 130 (80) | 251 (80) |
| Used 11−15 days | 9 (6) | 15 (9) | 24 (8) |
| Used more than 15 days | 4 (3) | 5 (3) | 9 (3) |
| Used (duration not specified) | 2 (1) | 0 | 2 (1) |
| Administration of placebo or *C. parvum* | | | |
| Not given | 18 (12) | 8 (5) | 26 (8) |
| Given 1−5 days postoperativ | 4 (3) | 6 (4) | 10 (3) |
| Given 6−10 days postoperativ | 115 (76) | 125 (77) | 240 (76) |
| Given 11−15 days postoperativ | 9 (6) | 19 (12) | 28 (9) |
| Given after 15th day postoperativ | 4 (3) | 4 (3) | 8 (3) |
| Unknown | 1 (1) | 1 (1) | 2 (1) |

[a] Includes sleeve resections, wedge resections, and combinations

**Table 7.** Worst degree of complication by treatment

|  | Worst degree of complication | | | |
|---|---|---|---|---|
|  | None | Mild | Moderate | Severe |
| Surgery plus placebo | 75 (50%) | 26 (17%) | 33 (22%) | 17 (11%) |
| Surgery plus *C. parvum* | 37 (23%) | 25 (15%) | 66 (41%) | 35 (22%) |

**Table 8.** Worst degree of complication by treatment after eliminating cases where placebo or *C. parvum* was not given

|  | Worst degree of complication | | | |
|---|---|---|---|---|
|  | None | Mild | Moderate | Severe |
| Surgery plus placebo | 69 (52%) | 23 (17%) | 27 (20%) | 14 (11%) |
| Surgery plus *C. parvum* | 34 (22%) | 21 (14%) | 65 (42%) | 35 (23%) |

**Table 9.** Complication by type and degree

|  | Surgery plus placebo | | |
|---|---|---|---|
|  | Mild | Moderate | Severe |
| Fever[a] | 15 | 13 | 1 |
| Nausea | 11 | 3 | 3 |
| Headache | 7 | 5 | 4 |
| Blood pressure change | 5 | 4 | 2 |
| Infection | 11 | 5 | 3 |
| Other | 10 | 22 | 8 |

|  | Surgery plus *C. parvum* | | |
|---|---|---|---|
|  | Mild | Moderate | Severe |
| Fever[a] | 35 | 48 | 13 |
| Nausea | 18 | 9 | 3 |
| Headache | 18 | 12 | 2 |
| Blood pressure change | 13 | 8 | 0 |
| Infection | 16 | 6 | 1 |
| Other | 13 | 26 | 24 |

[a] The degree of fever complication is standardized on the study forms as follows:

| | |
|---|---|
| Mild fever | $37.5° - 38°$ C |
| Moderate fever | $> 38°$ C |
| Severe | $> 40°$ C, severe with chills |
| Life-threatening | Fever with hypotension |

More severe complications were reported for the patients assigned to *C. parvum* ($p = 0.011$). If the patients who did not receive placebo or *C. parvum* are eliminated, this result is still  true ($p = 0.005$). The comparison of worst degree of complication where patients who did not receive placebo (18 cases) or *C. parvum* (8 cases) have been eliminated is given in Table 8.

The distribution of complications by type and degree for the two treatment regimens is given in Table 9. It is evident that there are more complications for patients receiving *C. parvum*. The severe "other" complications are listed in Table 10. The important factors appears to be fever and pleuritic or chest pain complications.

**Table 10.** Severe "Other" complications by treatment

| Complications | Number of patients experiencing a severe degree |
|---|---|
| Surgery plus placebo | |
| Pleuritic or chest pain | 4 |
| Dyspnea | 2 |
| Loss of appetite | 1 |
| Empyema | 1 |
| | |
| Surgery plus *C. parvum* | |
| Pleuritic or chest pain | 13[a] |
| Pleural exudate or effusion | 3 |
| An allergic reaction plus exanthem and pain | 1 |
| Asthma, respiratory insufficiency | 1 |
| Severe paralysis, right side | 1 |
| Postoperative hemothorax | 1 |
| Severe bleeding postoperative due to gastric ulcer | 1 |
| Severe cough | 1 |
| Severe pain (arm) | 1 |
| Severe pleural reaction | 1 |

[a] In conjunction with severe dyspnea in three cases

**Table 11.** Initial and post-treatment median blood values[a]

| | Surgery plus placebo (%) | Surgery plus *C. parvum* (%) |
|---|---|---|
| Initial WBC | 7,250 (148) | 7,500 (161) |
| Initial platelets | 265,000 (111) | 257,500 (120) |
| Initial monocytes | 310 (131) | 361 (138) |
| Post-treatment WBC | 9,150 (134) | 12,300 (147) |
| Post-treatment platelets | 365,500 (118) | 348,500 (126) |
| Post-treatment monocytes | 475 (118) | 560 (131) |

[a] The numbers given in parentheses give the number of patients with reported values

**Blood Components**

Initial WBC, platelet, and monocyte values are available for 98%, 74%, and 86% of the patients, respectively. Corresponding values for WBC, platelets, and monocytes following treatment are available for 89%, 78%, and 79% of the patients. The median counts for both the initial and post-treatment WBC, platelets, and monocytes are given in Table 11.

The distribution of patients by percentage increase in WBC and monocytes is given in Tables 12 and 13 respectively. Either the initial or post-treatment measurement is missing in 37 cases for the WBC and in 98 cases for monocytes. More than a 50% increase in WBC is observed in 59% of the patients assigned to *C. parvum* as opposed to 30% of the patients assigned to placebo ($p < 0.001$). The similar comparison for monocytes is 54% for *C. parvum* patients and 43% for placebo patients ($p = 0.065$).


**Disease-Free Interval**

The disease-free interval is measured from the date of resection until the date of recurrence of disease. If the patient died without evidence of disease, then death is still considered a failure of treatment unless it had no connection with the physical health of the individual. For example, one individual on the study committed suicide; his death will not be counted as a failure for either the evaluation of disease-free interval or survival. Seventeen patients were last reported without objective evidence of disease prior to death. These cases will be counted as failures as of the time of death.


**Table 12.** Percentage increase in WBC by treatment

|  | Surgery plus placebo (%) | Surgery plus *C. parvum* (%) |
|---|---|---|
| Less than 20% increase | 58 (44) | 32 (22) |
| 20%–50% increase | 34 (26) | 28 (19) |
| 50%–100% increase | 29 (22) | 39 (27) |
| Greater than 100% increase | 11 ( 8) | 46 (32) |
| Total | 132 (100) | 145 (100) |


**Table 13.** Percentage increase in monocytes by treatment

|  | Surgery plus placebo (%) | Surgery plus *C. parvum* (%) |
|---|---|---|
| Less than 20% increase | 47 (46) | 42 (37) |
| 20%–50% increase | 11 (11) | 10 ( 9) |
| 50%–100% increase | 5 ( 5) | 23 (20) |
| Greater than 100% increase | 39 (38) | 39 (34) |
| Total | 102 (100) | 114 (100) |

It is early to make any definitive comparisons of the treatments because only 18% (58 of 314) of the patients have "failed". However, it is possible to tentatively identify a few high-risk groups.

Figs. 3–9 present comparisons of treatment, surgical stage, participant histology, type of resection, type of bilobectomy, central histologic differentiation, and fever, with respect to disease-free interval.

Preliminary indications, tested by the log rank statistic, are that surgical stage ($p = 0.003$), type of resection ($p = 0.037$), and degree of differentiation ($p = 0.033$)

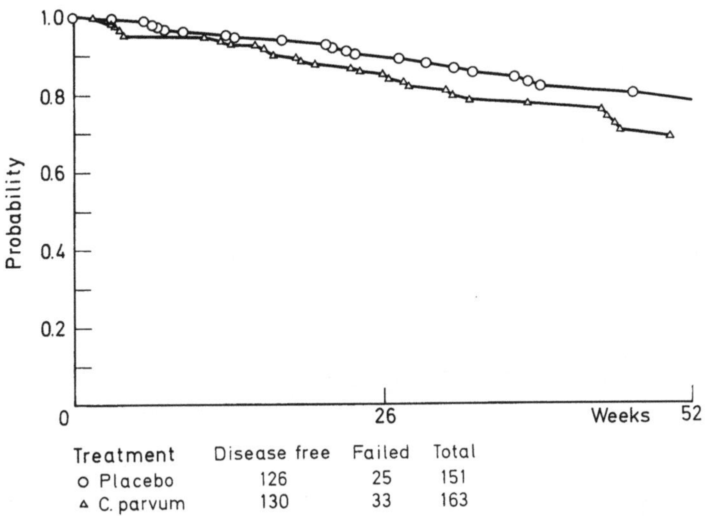



**Fig. 3.** Disease-free interval by treatment

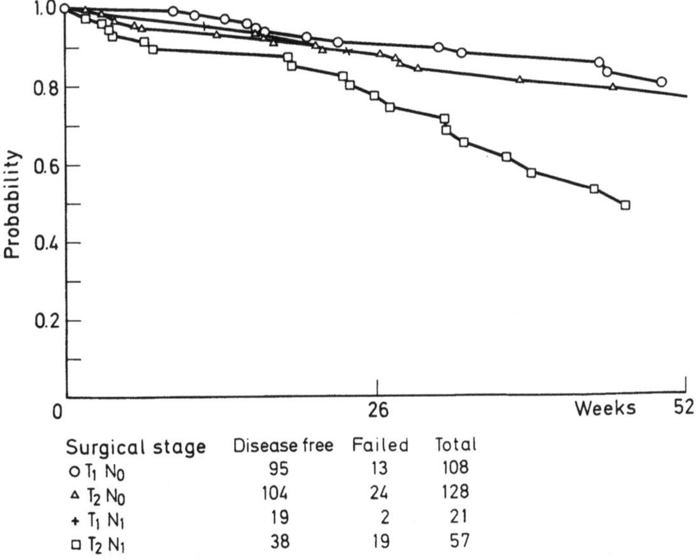



**Fig. 4.** Disease-free interval by surgical stage

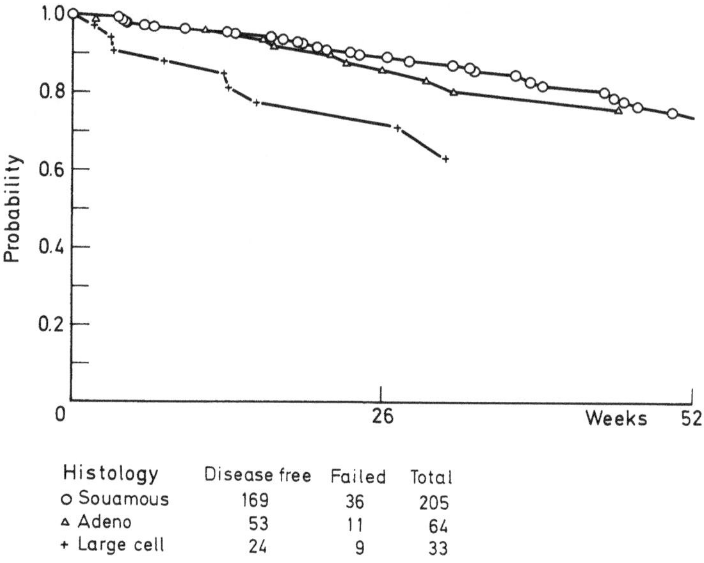



**Fig. 5.** Disease-free interval by participant histology

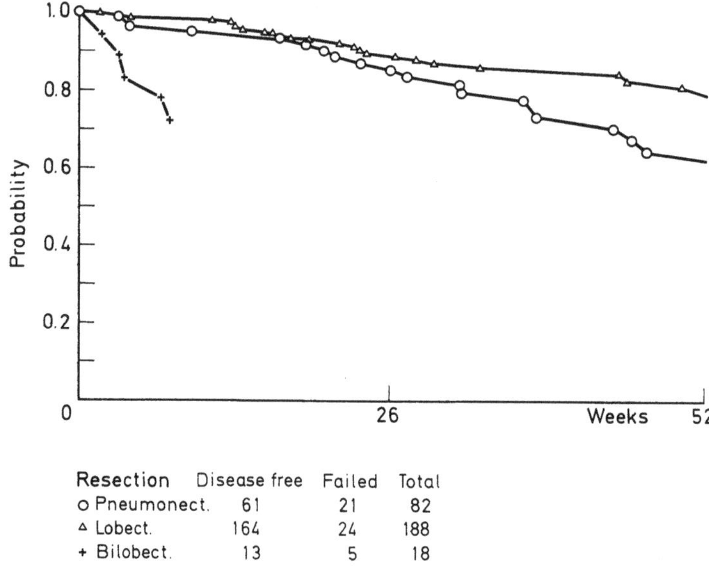



**Fig. 6.** Disease-free interval by type of resection

are prognostic factors. It appears that patients with a bilobectomy form a high-risk group.
Considering the bilobectomy patients, a comparison according to the unresected lobe is given in Fig. 7. This suggests that bilobectomy patients with the lower lobe remaining are at a greater risk for recurrence of disease than patients with the upper lobe remaining after bilobectomy.

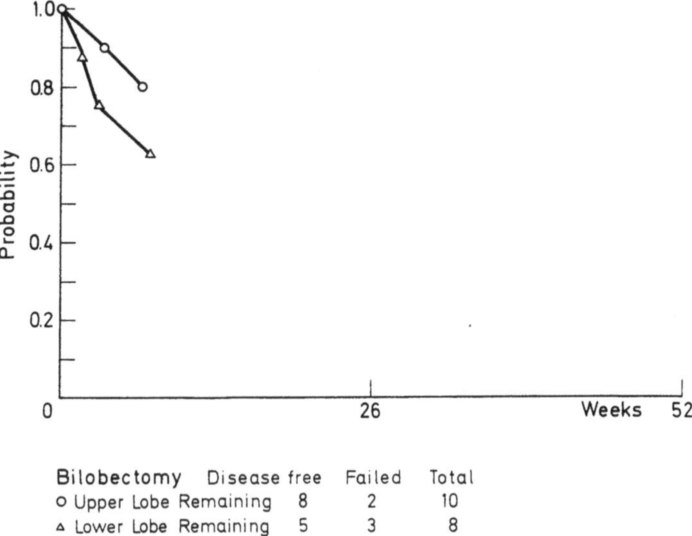



**Fig. 7.** Disease-free interval by type of bilobectomy

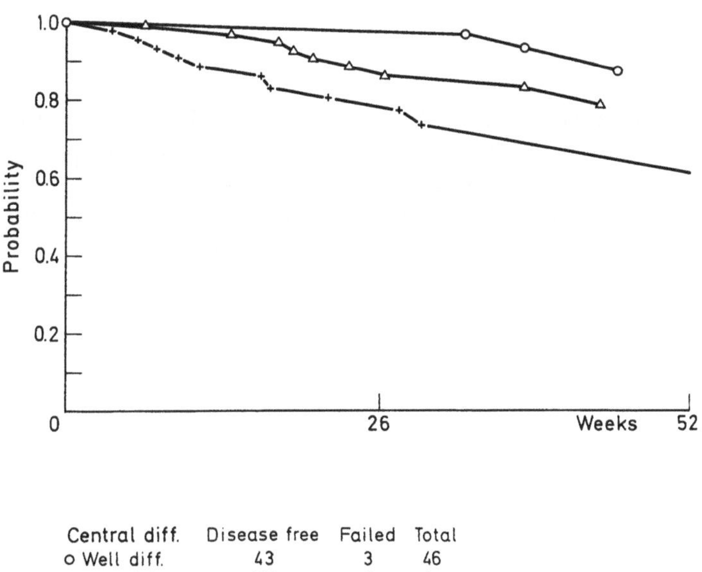



**Fig. 8.** Disease-free interval by central histologic differentiation

Central histology review is a very promising area and it is recommended that efforts be continued to gather and evaluate this material.

The relationship between fever and disease-free interval is depicted in Fig. 9 ($p = 0.03$). The disease-free interval appears to become shorter for patients experiencing a greater fever.

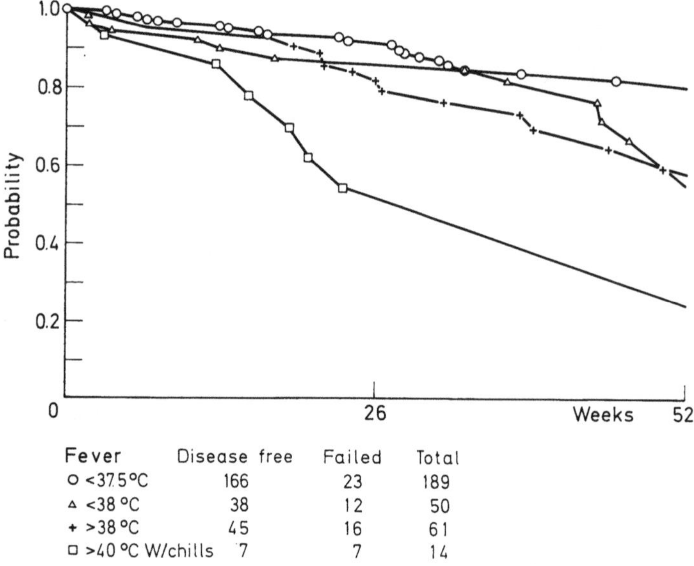


**Fig. 9.** Disease-free interval by observed fever post treatment

## Survival

Survival is measured from date of resection until death. It is too early to compare treatments because only 14% (45 of 314) of the patients have died.

The average follow-up time for the 314 analyzable cases is approximately 8 months. The factors of surgical stage, type of resection, and degree of differentiation which appear to be important with regard to disease-free interval also appear to be important prognostic factors for survival.

*Appendix 11. Terminology*

Clinical Trial

Investigation conducted on humans to evaluate some therapeutic program with respect to effectiveness, benefits and risks.

Clinic Sequence Number

The patient identification number assigned within each institution.

Data Manager

*Institution:* the individual responsible for collection and accurate and prompt reporting of data required in a study.
*Statistical Center:* the individual responsible for (1) reviewing the data for consistency and accuracy and unusual toxicity, (2) communicating with the institutions concerning missing or questionable data, (3) computer entry of data.

Disease Stage

A description of the extent of disease and involvement according to standardized classification.

End Points

Objective measures by which treatments are judged; such as survival, disease-free interval, and complications of treatment.

Collaborative Clinical Trial

Multi-participant clinical trial.

Follow-up

A term used to describe subsequent observations and reports in the reaction of a patient to therapy and status of that patient's disease.

Lost to Follow-up

A term used to describe the complete loss of contact with a patient.

Protocol

The written document to conduct the clinical trial.

Randomization

Random assignment to a treatment group by statistical design.

## Randomization Number

The sequential number assigned by the Operations Office when a patient is entered on a study. This number is used on all further correspondence concerning that patient.

## Statistician

An individual with statistical training who (1) collaborates in the design of the study and the forms, (2) designs the mechanism for allocating patients to the different arms of the study (in this case, randomization), and (3) analyzes the study data, i.e., calculates the success rates for the various treatment arms and adjusts for any imbalances so that comparisons are fair.

## Stratification

Proportionate grouping of patients into different prognostic categories to ensure that these prognostic factors do not imbalance the treatment comparisons.

## Study Coordinator

A physician in charge of a study with responsibility for: (1) planning the protocol, (2) monitoring possible side effects of treatment, and (3) making final decision on questionable cases.

# *Subject Index*

# Recent Results in Cancer Research

Sponsored by the Swiss League against Cancer. Editor in Chief: P. Rentchnick, Genève

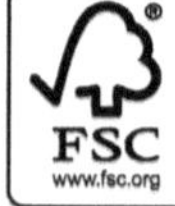



If you have any concerns about our products,
you can contact us on
ProductSafety@springernature.com

In case Publisher is established outside the EU,
the EU authorized representative is:
**Springer Nature Customer Service Center GmbH**
**Europaplatz 3, 69115 Heidelberg, Germany**

Printed by Libri Plureos GmbH
in Hamburg, Germany